Occupational Health Nursing

Edited by Brenda Slaney

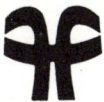

CROOM HELM LONDON

©1980 B.M. Slaney
Croom Helm Ltd, 2-10 St John's Road, London SW11

British Library Cataloguing in Publication Data
Occupational health nursing.
   1. Industrial nursing
   I. Slaney, Brenda
   610.73'46   RC966

   ISBN 0-85664-779-9

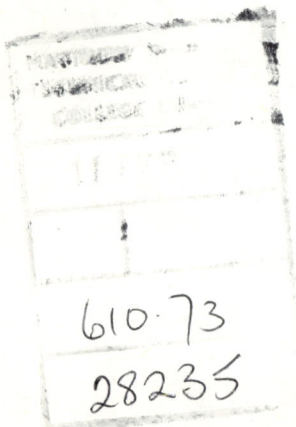

Printed in Great Britain by
Biddles Ltd, Guildford, Surrey

CONTENTS

PREFACE

The speciality of occupational health nursing is only just beginning to be recognised by the nursing profession and the general public, although nurses have been doing the job for over one hundred years. One of the reasons for this slow growth is possibly the lack of books upon the subject, and it is hoped that this book might begin to make good this gap in nursing literature.

This book, whose contributors are either practising occupational health nurses or occupational health nurse teachers, is a series of essays on some aspects of occupational health nursing. The topics were chosen from among those areas where occupational health nursing differs from general nursing and therefore was more difficult to comprehend. It is by no means comprehensive.

Although we are aware of the Sex Discrimination Act, the majority of nurses are female and therefore in the interests of an easy flow of language, the words 'she' and 'her' have been used to refer to any nurse, whether male or female: to balance this, the male pronouns 'he' and 'him' refer to doctors, workers, and patients. For the sake of brevity also, those who seek any sort of help from the nurse are 'patients' although we are aware that some people prefer the word 'client' particularly in the chapters on counselling and co-operation where it is, in fact sometimes used.

My thanks as editor go out to all the contributors who have co-operated so willingly in this project, and particularly to those who have helped in the scrutiny of the scripts and made many useful suggestions.

Brenda Slaney
April 1979

1 CONCEPTS OF OCCUPATIONAL HEALTH NURSING

Brenda Slaney

Some time ago, an experienced and qualified occupational health nurse arrived at a big engineering plant, to take up a new appointment to initiate and develop an Occupational Health Service. She was escorted to the room from which she was to start work by a member of senior management and observed by many eyes; she was, by her dress, instantly recognisable as a nurse. The room had formerly been used for First Aid work but had fallen into disuse: equipment was rather less than the statutory factory First Aid standard.[1] Within five minutes of the arrival of the nurse, a man, supported by a' workmate, staggered in; he was holding his left hand which was cruelly mutilated. The nurse at once applied a large First Aid dressing (which she had had the foresight to bring with her), summoned an ambulance, wrote a letter to the Accident Department and despatched the man to hospital. She then went into the plant to talk to the man's foreman and workmates to try to ascertain the circumstances surrounding the accident and how it could have been prevented. She found that there was no guard on the machine, there was no safety officer in the factory. The floor of the factory was thick with grease, machines were grossly crowded together; hot oil mist drenched the air as ventilation was totally inadequate and the injured man himself, over six feet in height, spent most of his working day bent nearly double in order to work the small-sized machine which drilled holes in thousands of small components each working day.

In this short story may be traced many of the concepts which underlie modern occupational health nursing. Some people have asked 'Is this work which nurses do in work places, where people are supposed to be well, nursing at all?' But here reference may be made to the functions of nursing personnel as set out in the World Health Organisation Technical Report no. 24 which states that the functions of nursing personnel are seen to be:

1. carrying out the therapeutic programme designed by physicians for sick patients including personal services aimed at hygiene and comfort;

2. maintenance of the physical and psychological environment conducive to recovery and health;

3. engaging the patient and his family in his recovery and rehabilitation;

4. instructing people, sick and well, in measures promoting total health (physical and mental) in a positive sense;

5. carrying out measures for the prevention of disease;

6. co-ordinating nursing efforts with other members of the health team and other members of community groups.[2]

About the same time a Joint Committee of the International Labour Organisation (ILO) and World Health Organisation (WHO)[3] used the term 'occupational health' for the first time and agreed that

occupational health should aim at:

1. the promotion and maintenance of the highest degree of physical, mental and social well-being of workers in all occupations;

2. the prevention amongst workers of departures from health caused by their working conditions;

3. the protection of workers in their employment from risks resulting from factors adverse to health;

4. the placing and maintenance of the worker in an occupational environment adapted to his physiological and psychological equipment, and to summarise: the adaptation of work to man and of each man to his job.

Furthermore, this same report states: 'occupational health carries out certain functions in regard to the health of workers, which are not appropriate to and could not be performed within the framework of personal medical care.'

Nurses working in industry and commerce across the world read these reports with interest and in effect said 'Yes, that is what we have been doing for years!' Nurses *are* engaged in trying to promote good health amongst all workers; this is done by assessing the health of individuals as they present themselves for the job, and in recommending that they are employed in a job suitable to their physical and (as far as possible) mental requirements. This will involve not only knowledge of health assessment but also of the physical and mental requirements of the job and the specific environment in which it is carried out, and not only at the time of first entry to the job but throughout a working life time. Sometimes specific measures have to be taken to protect workers from 'risks resulting from factors adverse to health', 'carrying out measures for the prevention of disease' and, all the time, people (sick and well) need instruction in promoting good health. These functions cannot be done in isolation but in co-operation with others.

If health is broken down by illness or injury, then the occupational health nurse usually works to standing orders agreed with the occupational physician as to what treatment is to be given. In the United Kingdom, treatment other than First Aid is usually agreed with the individual's own medical practitioner ('carrying out the therapeutic programme') so that there is wide variation on what treatment is actually carried out by the occupational health nurse in an enterprise and, at what stage the patient is passed to the care of the district nurse or hospital team, thus 'co-ordinating with other members of the health team and community groups'. But such episodes of absence from work are usually only very short incidents (although they may be very dramatic) in a working life and the occupational health nurse should play a most important part in the rehabilitation and resettlement 'engaging the patient and his family in his recovery and rehabilitation'.

A second joint ILO/WHO committee on Occupational Health was convened in Geneva in 1952.[4] In its report it stated:

The nurse has a key role in implementing all activities designed to promote the health of the worker. The precise duties of the industrial nurse depend on the general state of development of industrial health services in a plant or region or country. In general, the trained nurse has duties along the following lines:

1. assistance in general administration, maintenance and arrangement of health facilities in the plant;

2. emergency and primary treatment of accidents and illnesses based on standing orders from physicians;

3. assistance with pre-placement and other medical examinations;

4. arranging follow-up treatment, where indicated, including health supervision of employees returning to work after illness;

5. assistance in general preventive health measures in the plant;

6. health education and counselling;

7. assistance in supervision of factory hygiene and accident prevention;

8. advice on specific health questions to management and

workers;

9. maintenance of records and statistics; and

10. co-operation with, and referral of workers to, general community agencies for help, as necessary.

Among other recommendations it was suggested that the nurse should have direct access to top management.

It was with these functions in mind that a joint ILO/WHO seminar on the Nurse in Industry was organised in London in April 1957.[5] The meeting was preceded by the circulation to the participants of a selected bibliography, a background paper and a questionnaire. The outcome of this seminar was that it largely confirmed the views of the work of the nurse as had been put forward in the 1952 report, but it stated that variation was influenced by the country and the enterprise in which the nurse was working, the existence or absence of other health services and the status of nursing (including general education) in that country.

Prior to this date (1957) nurses had been excluded from membership of the Permanent Commission and International Association on Occupational Health. This organisation, founded by Professor Luigi Carozzi in 1906 in Milan, had always been a society of physicians, meeting on a triennial basis (apart from war years); but in 1948 industrial nurses, realising that they were making a great contribution to occupational health, resolved to work for the right of full membership of the Commission. This was not granted until 1957 in Helsinki, when Mrs Gwen Doherty of the United Kingdom, Miss Ruth Säynäjarvi of Finland and Miss Sara Wagner of the United States were elected. Nine years later, the Council of the Commission further recognised the work of the nurses when a nursing committee, to study the nurse's contribution to the health of the worker, was appointed. The committee under the chairmanship of Miss Mary Blakeley of the United Kingdom, set to work at once and published its first report in 1969.[6] The report was based on the answers to a questionnaire which had been circulated to 70 countries, that is 63 countries whose nurses were in communication with the International Council of Nurses, and, where there was no national nursing association, to 7 other countries where there was a doctor member of the Permanent Commission.

The report showed that, in the industrially developed countries, nurses, to a greater or lesser degree, *were* carrying out the work described in the Report of 1952. In other countries Occupational

Health Services were beginning, and starting to employ nurses. During the time that this report was being composed (1968) a seminar had been convened by ILO/WHO in Geneva on the work of the occupational health nurse. The key background paper was written by Miss Vera Stoves of the United Kingdom.[7]

An entry appeared in the International Standard Classification of Occupations.[8]

0. 71. 40.

Occupational Health Nurse

Provides professional nursing services and health information for employees in work places; gives first aid treatment at places of employment for injuries and illnesses and arranges for further medical care, if necessary; renews surgical dressings and gives other routine treatment for minor injuries or disorders at work place or patient's home; gives inoculations, assists with health examinations; keeps records of persons treated and prepares reports for use in compensation claims and for other purposes; informs employer concerning health problems among the employees; provides health and hygiene information to workers.

About the same time (1965-9) in the United States of America, Miss Marjorie Keller, the Assistant Professor of Nursing and Principal Investigator of the University of Tennessee College of Nursing, was working on a project to identify the occupational health nursing content essential in baccalaureate education for professional nursing.[9] She first reviewed the relevant literature in education, nursing and occupational health nursing; she then developed a theoretical framework consisting of an integration of the work of Leavell and Clark on the levels-of-prevention approach to health care and the work of Maslow on the hierarchy-of-needs professional theory.

H.R. Leavell and E.G. Clark in their book *Preventive Medicine for the Doctor in his Community: an Epidemiological Approach*[10] had identified three levels of preventive medicine: primary (health promotion and specific protection), secondary (early diagnosis, prompt treatment and disability limitation) and tertiary (rehabilitation). On the other hand, A.H. Maslow in his work *Motivation and Personality*,[11] identified six basic human needs: physiological, safety or protection, love and belongingness, esteem, self-actualisation and aesthetic. In Keller's study the aesthetic needs were not considered as there was insufficient time to explore them. Keller brought these two theories together and formed a framework covering 25 categories. Although this approach was developed for occupational health nursing, it was sufficiently broad to form a framework for all nursing. The importance of this work was that, for the first time, a theoretical basis for occupational health nursing was suggested.

A second report of the Nursing Committee of the Permanent Commission and International Association, published in 1973, used this theoretical basis to discuss the education needed for occupational health nursing, after general nurse training.[12]

These nursing reports collectively show the concern of the occupational health nurse for the 'whole' person who presents for work: the basic needs of the person are shown against the total health situation. This is not to say that the occupational health nurse alone delivers total health care in every part; this is where teamwork (as discussed in Chapter 9 of this book) is important. But the occupational health nurse at work can show this total concern for the health of people. This is in contrast to those practitioners (of many disciplines) who identify occupational health entirely with those diseases or injuries which occur during or directly arising out of the occupation. Such work is, of course, essential and the nurse can play an important part in it, but for most nurses it is not the whole concept of occupational health. For example, in Great Britain in 1976, in the employed population over 300 million working days were lost due to sickness absence from work,[13] whilst there were only 2 million working days lost due to industrial poisonings and 18 million working days lost due to notifiable industrial accident. (An accident is notifiable when it causes loss of life to a person employed in a factory or disables any such person for more than three days from earning full wages at his work.) The small number of days lost due to industrial disease and accident is due to constant vigilance by everyone interested in occupational health: government, legislators, employers and employees, designers, inspectors as well as the specialist occupational health workers. However, most occupational health nurses are also greatly interested in the concept of the well person, in trying to prevent unnecessary suffering and illness and, in effect, making a contribution towards achieving total health in the working population and thus doing something towards reducing the enormous figure of 300 million working days lost attributed to illness.

This wider view of occupational health was apparently in the minds of an expert committee of the World Health Organisation in 1973, when in a report entitled 'Environmental and Health Monitoring in

Occupational Health'[14] they wrote, 'Even in highly industrialised countries the occurrence of occupational diseases is still too high and additional health problems affecting the gainfully employed include chronic noncommunicable diseases, mental disorders, alcoholism and drug abuse.' The report also states, 'Occupational health monitoring offers opportunities of developing a better understanding of the chronic degenerative diseases and of the diseases of special concern to ageing people.' Earlier in the report they also noted that in developing countries the prevalence of communicable diseases was sometimes higher among occupational groups than in the general population.

This same report had given a new statement of the objectives of an occupational health programme.

An occupational health programme aims to promote and maintain the highest possible level of health among the gainfully employed upon whom the economic welfare of the community depends. To meet these objectives it is necessary:

1. to identify and bring under control at the work place all chemical, physical, mechanical, biological and psychosocial agents that are known to be or suspected of being hazardous;

2. to ensure that the physical and mental demands imposed on people at work by their respective jobs are properly matched with their individual anatomical, physiological and psychological capabilities, needs and limitations.

3. to provide effective measures to protect those who are especially vulnerable to adverse working conditions.

The report spoke of the need for continuous monitoring of health, and in this the nurse can make a most valuable contribution. The nurse can play a part in the early detection of occupational disease not previously recognised. She may be the first to realise that a number of employees who have reported with similar symptoms may all have worked in the same department, or may be from different departments but all have been in contact with a certain substance. The nurse's vigilance is also important in revealing other sources of health risk, especially those associated with stress. These risks do not cause identifiable occupational disease, but are thought to increase psycho-biological vulnerability and possibly contribute to general ill health.

How far are these concepts reflected in modern occupational health nursing? An examination of the literature of the last ten years is indicative of trends.

In a report of a conference held in Bulgaria in 1971[15] a Bulgarian
nurse mentioned a training course:

> the curriculum varies but it is mainly on the preventive aspects of
> the work (i.e. of occupational health nursing): the nurses are taught
> about the various influences of the industrial environment on the
> health of the worker and on the problems of the pregnant woman at
> work. Some training is given too on the investigation of
> cardiovascular, respiratory and metabolic disturbances.
> Recommendations are given to the nurses about improving working
> conditions and about participation in social problems.

Given that the training is preparing people to do a job, this is some
indication of what occupational health nurses in Bulgaria are doing.

Gail Frische co-authored an article on occupational health nursing
for the New Zealand Nursing Journal in March 1975,[16] and described
her work as follows:

> diagnosis and treatment of work/non-work injuries;
> diagnosis and treatment of illnesses;
> treatment of medical emergencies occurring at work;
> provision of immunisation;
> health interviews of apparently well people;
> selective screening lists on workers exposed to specific hazards;
> provision of a counselling service;
> rehabilitation of people following injury, illness or operation;
> home and hospital visiting of injured or ill workers;
> assistance with family problems where they are affecting the work
>   situation;
> participation on committees planning new developments, new
>   processes or new plants;
> concern with the cleanliness of amenities and eating facilities;
> provision of health education in relation to work hazards and
>   general living;
> participation on safety committees at work;
> knowledge of fundamental hazards at work.

She also said in the same article:

> Health services at work are fundamentally different from traditional
> general practitioner services in that they combine treatment and

prevention, social work and rehabilitation, are free to the person needing them, waiting time is minimal as is travelling distance to the service and most importantly, the service is based around the nurse rather than the doctor.

A month later the Philippine Journal of Nursing reported a panel discussion of nurses in which Zylma Sanchez represented the nurse in industry.[17] She said that the major objective of an occupational health nursing service was to provide an adequate programme for employees which would help them maintain the highest potential level of health and efficiency. The functions outlined reflected all the work known to occupational health nurses in previous reports. She concluded her remarks by saying that there was every indication that the services of professional nurses would be increasingly used by industry and that nurses would assume an ever widening range of responsibilities.

The contribution of Scandinavian nurses to the development of occupational health nursing is a very important one, but most of their writings are inaccessible. Ruth Säynäjarvi, however, who was one of the first three nurses accepted into the Permanent Commission in 1957, made an important speech in Brighton, England, in 1975. In it she showed that her colleagues in Scandinavia, whilst carrying out all the commonly accepted functions of the occupational health nurse, are developing their interest and knowledge in ergonomics and the posture of people at work. These studies have been carried out among such varied occupations as librarians and car and construction workers.[18]

The nursing process was first described by F.G. Abdellah in the USA in 1960,[19] but it does not appear to have been explicitly applied to occupational health nursing until July 1975, when the Department of Environmental Health of the University of Cincinnati published a book entitled *Standards, Interpretations and Audit Criteria for Performance of Occupational Health Programs.*[20] Again Maslow's hierarchy of needs was used in identifying universal human needs in a nursing situation. But this time it was used against the background of general systems analysis.

In a paper presented to the 34th Annual Meeting of the American Association of Industrial Nurses Inc., in Cincinnati in April 1976, Miss Cahall,[21] the Assistant Professor of the University there, described the use of the nursing process in the industrial setting. She showed that nurses must think in the cyclical terms of assessing, planning, intervening and evaluating.

She spoke at length of the need for a complete data base about the

worker before assessment could be made and from which the nursing
plan could be designed, the intervention carried out and later
evaluation made to ascertain if the plan was successful. She gave six
criteria to be used in evaluating nursing care:

1. Is the plan of nursing care co-ordinated with the plan of
medical care?
2. Is it based on scientific principles and is it therapeutically
effective?
3. Does it ensure maximum physical and emotional safety and
security for the worker?
4. Does it reflect immediate and long range planning to help the
worker regain or maintain the highest level of wellness possible?
5. Does it meet psychosocial and physiological needs and
recognise the inter-relatedness of these needs?
6. Does the plan of nursing care provide for the maximum
amount of family participation?

At the same conference Carol Silverstein,[22] another member of the
University staff, demonstrated a practical example of how the nursing
care plan was used (see Figure 1.1).

The nursing care plan is essentially one to encourage a plan of care
for the worker taking into consideration everything which affects his
well-being. Occupational health nurses are usually working with the
same people for longer periods than most of their nursing colleagues
and should, therefore, be in a better position to work through the whole
process, evaluating and adjusting all the time. Both Cahall and
Silverstein seem to be applying the nursing process to the care of an
individual, yet an occupational health nurse should also be applying
the system to groups of people under her care. A way in which this
might be done is suggested in the paper by Tinkham[23] 'The Plant as
the Patient of the Occupational Health Nurse'.

The occupational health nurse must study the epidemiology of
groups of people under her care, to try to discover trends and to take
appropriate action. Such observation was surely in the mind of Yukiko
Okui of Japan, when she wrote 'Japanese law requires the employer to
conduct periodical health examinations, at least once a year, for
employees. Such legislative action was realised in conjunction with the
prevention, early detection and treatment of the rampant pulmonary
tuberculosis, the control of which had once been the major issue in the
health administration of the country.'[24]

Figure 1.1: Detailed Nursing Care Plan

NAME: John Doe   AGE: 46   WORK LOCATION: Foundry

SEX: Male   RACE: Oriental   WORK EXPOSURE: Silica

HEALTH SUMMARY: Normal healthy male, wt 220#, no acute illnesses, family history of diabetes & tuberculosis. No work limitations.

Date	Problem	Approach	Date of solution
	I. Work exposure to silica	1. Ask industrial hygienist what the exposure level is in this work area.	
		2. If the TLV is exceeded see what dust control methods are being implemented.	
		3. Encourage yearly physical with x-ray.	
		4. Teaching program for personal hygiene.	
	II. Overweight	1. Encourage to diet sensibly	
		2. Help plan diet.	
		3. Encourage to check wt. at scales in medical unit weekly.	
	III. Family history of diabetes	1. Teach symptoms of diab.	
		2. Encourage yr. physical	
	IV. Teenage son on drugs	1. Suggested he: a) contact local M.D. b) seek help from local drug abuse program.	
	V. Change in work location- exposures include lead	1. Establish a specific time interval for urine and blood leads with MD	
		2. Instruct in personal hygiene measures.	

A review of some articles which have appeared recently in the English press, shows how diverse are the situations in which occupational health nursing takes place: 'Racecourse Nurses',[25] 'Work of an Occupational Health Nurse in a Motor Company',[26] 'Rehabilitation: the Nurse's Role; Occupational Health Nurses' Work at the Central Electricity Generating Board',[27] 'Post Office Nursing',[28] 'Nursing on a Cruise Ship',[29] 'Industrial Nursing at the Royal Mint',[30] 'Focus on Care of the Men Who Cut Coal',[31] 'Nursing in Fleet Street',[32] 'Is Your Service really Necessary?'[33] (in hospital) and so on. Throughout all these articles runs the common core of occupational health nursing, some types of work demanding an emphasis on one aspect and some on another.

Most recently, occupational health nursing has been discussed in Parliament. [34] Mr Hodgson, Member of Parliament for Walsall (North) said 'The need for properly adapted work, for giving advice on suitable jobs and for providing initial treatment is and will continue to be of vital importance in ensuring that British Industry is as effective as possible and that people do the jobs they find most enjoyable and for which they are best trained and best suited temperamentally. The occupational health nurses have a vital role to play.'

So, to return to the story with which this chapter opened. The situation can be interpreted as a 'simple' case needing first aid treatment, or it can be interpreted, as a total situation, of a type, around and through which concepts of occupational health nursing have been developing for over a hundred years.

Notes

1. Factories Act 1961, First Aid Regulations (HMSO, London).
2. World Health Organisation, Technical Report no.24 (Geneva, 1950), p.5.
3. World Health Organisation, Occupational Health/2, unpublished document (Geneva, 1950).
4. International Labour Organisation Expert Committee on Occupational Health Second Report (Geneva, 1952).
5. World Health Organisation, Joint ILO/WHO Seminar on the Nurse in Industry (Regional Office for Europe, Copenhagen, 1957).
6. Permanent Commission and International Association on Occupational Health, Nursing Subcommittee, Report on the Nurse's Contribution to the Health of the Worker, 1966-9 (The Commission, 1969).
7. International Labour Office, *The Occupational Health Nurse*, pp.5-20, Occupational Safety and Health Series no.23 (Geneva, 1970).
8. International Labour Office, *International Standard Classification of Occupations*, Major group 0/1 Professional Technical and Related Workers (Geneva, 1969).
9. M.J. Keller and W.T. May, *Occupational Health Content in Baccalaureate*

Nursing Education (US Department of Health Education and Welfare, Cincinnati, Ohio, 1970).

10. H.R. Leavell and E.G. Clark, *Preventive Medicine for the Doctor in His Community: an Epidemiological Approach*, 3rd edn. (McGraw Hill Book Company, Blakistan Division, 1965).

11. A.H. Maslow, *Motivation and Personality* (Harper and Row, New York, 1954).

12. Permanent Commission and International Association on Occupational Health, Nursing Sub-committee, Report on the Nurse's Contribution to the Health of the Worker 1971-3, *Education of the Nurse* (The Commission, 1974).

13. Central Statistical Office and Central Office of Information, *Guide to Official Statistics* (HMSO, London, 1977).

14. World Health Organisation, 'Environmental and Health Monitoring in Occupational Health', Technical Report no.535 (WHO, Geneva, 1975).

15. M. French and M. Williams, 'Bulgarian Conference', *Occupational Health*, vol.24, no.1 (January 1972), p.14.

16. G.A. Frische and W.J. Glass, 'Occupational Health Nursing', *New Zealand Nursing Journal* (March 1975), pp.4-6.

17. Z. Sanchez, 'Unity in Diversity', *Philippine Journal of Nursing*, vol.XLIV, no.2 (1975), pp.82-4.

18. Permanent Commission and International Association on Occupational Health, 'Hur Kan Foretagsskoterskan Bidra med Atgarder for att uppna en god arbetsmiljo' (Sweden, 1975).

19. F.G. Abdellah *et al.*, *Patient Centred Approaches to Nursing* (Macmillan, New York, 1960).

20. Department of Environmental Health, *Standards, Interpretations and Audit Criteria for Performance of Occupational Health Programs* (University of Cincinnati, July 1975).

21. J.B. Cahall, 'The Use of the Nursing Process in the Industrial Setting', *Occupational Health Nursing*, vol.24, no.11 (November 1976), pp.9-13.

22. C. Silverstein, 'Implementing and Evaluating the Nursing Process in the Occupational Health Unit', *Occupational Health Nursing*, vol.24, no.11 (November 1976), pp.14-19.

23. C. Tinkham, 'The Plant as the Patient of the Occupational Health Nurse', *Nursing Clinics of North America*, vol.7, no.1 (March 1972).

24. Y. Okui, 'Health Counselling by the Occupational Health Nurse', XVIII International Congress Abstracts (The Commission, Brighton, England, 1975).

25. J. Cullinan, 'Racecourse Nurses', *Nursing Times*, vol.67 (21 January 1971), pp.69-71.

26. M. Haynes, 'Careers in Nursing. A Job with a Difference: Work of an Occupational Health Nurse in a Motor Company', *Nursing Times*, vol.67 (30 September 1971), pp.1215-17.

27. J. Manuel, 'Rehabilitation: the Nurse's Role; Occupational Health Nurses' Work at the Central Electricity Generating Board, Midlands Region', *Occupational Health*, vol.28, part.9 (September 1976), pp.418-19.

28. 'Post Office Nursing. A Day in the Life of. . .', *Nursing Mirror*, vol.140 (19 June 1975), pp.58-9.

29. 'Follow the Sun – the Nurse's Life Afloat. Nursing on a Cruise Ship', *Nursing Times*, vol.71 (16 January 1975), pp.92-3.

30. 'In the Money. Industrial Nursing at the Royal Mint', *Nursing Times*, vol.69 (1 March 1973), pp.289-91.

31. J. Richardson, 'Focus on Care of the Men Who Cut Coal', *Nursing Week*, no.13 (17 January 1974), pp.6-7.

32. V. Walter, 'Nursing in Fleet Street', *Evening Standard Nightingale*

Fellowship Journal, no.90 (January 1974), pp.528-9.
    33. V. Jones, 'Is Your Service really Necessary?' *Occupational Health,* vol.29, nos.11 and 12 (November, December 1977) and vol.30, no.1 (January 1978).
    34. House of Commons Parliamentary Debate Official Report. *Hansard,* 'Nurses, Midwives, Health Visitors Bill', Committee Stage, 7 December 1978, cols.179-88.

Further Reading

American Association of Occupational Health Nurses, *Objectives of an Occupational Health Nursing Service* (New York, 1977)

Australian Occupational Health Nurses Association, *Guidelines for the Employment of Occupational Health Nurses in Australia* (Sydney, 1978)

M.L. Brown, 'The Occupational Health Nurse: A New Perspective' in C. Zenz (ed.), *Occupational Medicine* (Year Book Medical Publishers, Chicago, 1975), pp.41-59

M.D. Green, 'Changing Attitudes (towards nursing, and in particular towards occupational health nursing)', *Occupational Health*, vol.24, no.5 (1974), pp.175-8.

D. Radwanski, 'Nursing and Occupational Health' in A. Ward Gardner (ed.), *Current Approaches to Occupational Medicine* (John Wainwright and Sons Ltd, Bristol, 1979), pp.218-29

D. Radwanski and J.C.H. Pearson, 'Occupational Health Nursing in Scotland', *Transactions of the Society of Occupational Medicine*, vol.22, no.4 (October, 1972), pp.122-5

Royal College of Nursing and National Council of Nurses of the United Kingdom, Occupational Health Section, '1952-1973: 21st Anniversary and Annual Conference at the Royal Society of Medicine, 23-24 November' (Rcn, London, 1973)

Second Australian Convention, Occupational Health Nursing: Focus on the Future (Sydney, 1976)

B. Slaney, 'The Need for Professional Identification in Occupational Health Nursing', *Occupational Health Nursing*, vol.21, no.5 (19 May 1973), p.33

H. Yura and M.B. Walsh, 'The Nursing Process; Assessing, Planning, Implementing and Evaluating', Proceedings of the Continuing Education Series conducted at the Catholic University of America (The University, Washington PC, 1967)

2 PROFESSIONAL RESPONSIBILITY AND ROLE DEVELOPMENT

P.V. Lloyd

Occupational health nursing is a challenging sphere of nursing practice, affording considerable professional satisfaction and opportunities for role development.

It is important for the nurse to be clear at the outset about the nature of the challenges that lie ahead, the role to be developed, and the means available to achieve these goals. Occupational health nursing is a developing speciality, which is founded on the traditional nursing role but embodies many additional skills. The ethics of nursing based on the concept of a caring profession, are well recognised in the occupational health field, although because the nurse may be professionally isolated, these ethics may be challenged from time to time.

The nurse in this speciality has every opportunity to enjoy independence of action and freedom to initiate and develop health care policies whilst working at times alongside other members of the occupational health professions. Nursing in this setting enables the individual nurse practitioner to exert influence among groups of workers in a wide range of occupations.

Educational Preparation

Any nurse contemplating a career in occupational health nursing should obtain additional training in occupational health practice. The Royal College of Nursing of the United Kingdom (Rcn), has been teaching nurses in the principles and practice of occupational health nursing since 1934, and such courses, geared to meet the needs of the modern nurse student, are being provided in increasing numbers today.

The nursing profession recognises the need to ensure that standards of competence to practise in specialised areas are established. The nurse entering occupational health nursing is no exception, and measures to bring about statutory control over the education and certification of occupational health nurses are clearly desirable.

The emphasis in occupational health nursing is placed upon the prevention of disease and injury arising from or through work activity. Since the syllabus and training requirements as well as the centres providing training courses, change from time to time, an up-to-date list of approved centres and other information relating to education in occupational health nursing may be obtained from the Director of Education, Royal College of Nursing.[1]

Knowledge and Training

Education and professional development are ongoing and complementary activities which should continue right throughout the nurse's professional career. Professional competence implies being professionally up-to-date at all times. The advantages of attending a professional course or conference are not only to be found in listening to lectures, but in meeting with and talking to other practitioners in the occupational health field.

At the Work Place

The time to establish a correct professional understanding and working relationship with the employer and his representatives is at the time of interview and prior to acceptance of a Contract of Employment. To start off at a disadvantage is a handicap which may take a lifetime to overcome. For this reason, the interview provides the nurse with the opportunity to establish the scope and responsibilities of the post, the functions to be undertaken, and the status, salary and conditions of work under which the occupational health nurse will be expected to operate.

The interviewer may not always be clear about the proper role and function of an Occupational Health Nursing Service, and if duties and responsibilities are suggested which have no bearing on this, the nurse should not accept the post unless changes can be negotiated which will allow the nurse to contribute her skills in an appropriate manner, for the maximum benefit of all employed in the undertaking.

The Personnel Department

There is a personnel function in most industries. One of the functions of personnel management is to ensure that provision is made to meet the employer's statutory duties in respect of the health, safety and welfare of the workers. The Institute of Personnel Management is the professional body which lays down conditions for the examination and membership into the Institute of Personnel Officers and higher personnel executives.

There are, in addition, personnel officers who are not qualified nor members of their own professional institute. The standards of personnel management are, therefore, likely to be variable.

The occupational health nurse invariably comes into regular contact with the staff of the Personnel Department because of the close interest both take in the individual worker. It is essential, therefore, to establish at the outset a close and harmonious working relationship with the Personnel Department staff, a relationship founded on a clear appreciation of the role of the occupational health nurse, which is quite separate from the role and function of the Personnel Officer.

Well defined lines of communication and administrative responsibility must be agreed. The occupational health nurse should ensure that the following principles are understood and agreed by both parties:

1. The Occupational Health Nursing Service should be seen to be quite separate from the Personnel Department.

2. Workers should always be able to approach the Occupational Health Centre without having to report first to the Personnel Department.

3. The Health Centre should be close to, but physically separated from, the Personnel Offices. If both activities are combined in one geographical area, separate entrances and waiting areas should be provided.

4. Occupational health nurses should not accept combined posts within the Personnel Office and Health Centre.

5. Employee health records maintained voluntarily by the Occupational Health Service should be completely confidential to the staff of the Occupational Health Service.

Managerial Accountability

The occupational health department, whether it is staffed by one nurse or a team of nurses and doctors, is a separate specialised functional department within the organisation. The senior occupational health practitioner should assume managerial control and responsibility for the smooth running of the occupational health department. This accountability should be to a senior member of the organisation's management structure after separate budgetary provision has been made.

Managerial responsibility for nursing affairs should be through the most senior nurse designated in charge of the Occupational Health Nursing Services. A link is also necessary with the organisation's Personnel function in respect of holiday entitlements, dispute and grievance procedures, salary and conditions of service, career and training, and any other employee relations activity to which the nurse as an employee would be entitled.

Professional Accountability

No occupational health nurse should be made professionally accountable to anyone other than to another nurse. It follows that the occupational health nurse is the professional adviser on occupational health nursing. The nurse will, therefore, offer professional advice to anyone in the organisation for whom the Occupational Health Service is being provided, including access to the highest level of manager within the organisation, appropriate in the circumstances — if a small organisation, to the Works Manager, or in a multi-national organisation, to a Director at Board level.

Professional advice should not only be offered at employer level, when the need has been established, but at every level within the organisation through the formal and informal lines of communication which the occupational health nurse should establish. The nurse, as a professional adviser, is also free to refer problems to outside agencies such as the Employment Medical Advisory Service for further advice and information. The employer and work representatives should whenever possible, be given prior warning if such action is contemplated, especially if this might bring the organisation into conflict with these authorities. The nurse should always remember that her role is to act as a professional adviser. Management should welcome and respect the nurse's advice and whenever possible, act upon it.

Trade Unions and Workers

Any confrontations between employers and their work people should not concern the occupational health nurse who needs to be very adept at playing a neutral role. The occupational health nurse has a responsibility to work with trade unions and especially their health and safety representatives, in order to assist in identifying and helping to eliminate health and safety problems. In this respect, the occupational health nurse is to be likened to the safety adviser.

The expectations of management and health and safety representatives should not be diametrically opposed, as both are required to work together to ensure a safe and healthy working environment. The differences lie in the approach to these problems and the methods used to achieve a satisfactory result. The occupational health nurse must be careful to give the same advice to either side and not appear to be seen to support a management or union position. For this reason, the occupational health nurse should ensure that she participates as an impartial adviser in any health and safety committee established at the work place.

The Occupational Health Nurse as a Trade Union Member

The occupational health nurse, as an employee, may wish to join or be obliged to join, because of an agreement between the management and certain trade unions, a recognised trade union at the place of work for negotiation purposes. Many occupational health nurses may prefer to belong to a combined professional organisation and trade union – the Royal College of Nursing (Rcn) is an appropriate organisation.

The nurse should be fully aware of the differences between a professional nursing trade union and an industrial trade union. Whilst the nurse's own professional organisation is able to identify with the nurse's needs, and represent these views to management, the employer may not accord recognition, although the views of the professional organisation and trade union carry considerable influence in establishing occupational health nursing grades and a salary structure.

It may be necessary for occupational health nurses to belong to a trade union in order to protect their economic and social interests. The occupational health nurse should inquire carefully before joining any trade union whether she would be required to participate in any industrial action, including strike action, which may be called by the trade union. Furthermore, inquiries should be made about the arrangements the union has made to provide the nurse with professional indemnity insurance to protect the nurse in the event of legal action being taken against her by an employee or even by their employer!

If the answers to these important questions are unsatisfactory, the occupational health nurse should look elsewhere for adequate safeguards. The Rcn provides indemnity insurance for each of its members and observes a code of ethics which never places the nurse in the position of putting patients at risk through strike action. Where recognition of the Rcn cannot be secured at the place of work for negotiation purposes, the occupational health nurse should consider very seriously joining both for the additional safeguards and benefits a nurse in active practice requires, especially whilst working in professional isolation.

Professional Organisation

A professional organisation is a corporate body which acts on behalf of its members and seeks to bring about change and influence events in the interests of the profession in general and its members in particular. The individual nurse, often professionally isolated as the only representative of the nursing profession in the organisation, has a responsibility to join and make a contribution to professional development and activity. Such organisations provide an opportunity for members to meet together to discuss matters of common interest. They also aim to assist members to increase their knowledge and enhance their contribution to nursing and strive to increase awareness within the profession generally of the expert contribution of occupational health nursing.

These objectives are met by providing conferences and courses, information through consultation, a committee structure and by way of working parties and informal meetings. The leaders of the organisation are likely to be elected from among members engaged in occupational health nursing as their principal sphere of nursing activity. It is clearly in the interests of the occupational health nurse to demonstrate professional awareness by playing an active role within the profession in order to meet the needs and aspirations of occupational health nurses wherever they work.

The employer should be made aware that the occupational health nurse has a responsibility to become involved with her own professional organisation and should be encouraged to allow leave of absence in order for the nurse to participate in professional activity.

Professional education and certification provide the foundation for competence to practise. However, the nurse requires other skills and personal qualities, in addition to professional training, in order to succeed in any given situation, especially when pioneering a new service.

Since the occupational health nurse may not be readily accepted by those with whom she will come into contact, skills of tact and perseverance, personality and ability to relate to people at all levels within the organisation are qualities which will need to be fully utilised if the nurse is to succeed.

The occupational health nurse has to strive to become an accepted figure, trusted and respected by all. This situation is not achieved automatically nor may it be demanded. The basis of the professionalism of nursing is based upon the knowledge and skills of the nurse. The nurse in a hospital environment must, of necessity, relate to her patients in a different way to an occupational health nurse who is, in effect, projecting a totally different image of nursing to the one the general public has come to accept.

The occupational health nurse ought to read professional nursing and medical publications regularly and ensure that other relevant reading material[2] is made available at the place of work and be costed in as a part of the occupational health department's budget.

Health Service and Other Agencies

The list of other people with whom the occupational health nurse comes into contact is wide and diverse. This situation is similar to that of the ward sister with day-to-day charge of the ward and who remains in control as the fulcrum around which all other services rotate.

In occupational health practice, the nurse is the one who provides continuity of care; she is the linchpin of reliability and the one who co-ordinates patient or client services. She must ensure that the people amongst whom she works are fully aware of the aims of the Occupational Health Service and the qualifications of its staff. Once professional people are aware of the type of Occupational Health Service provided and facilities and resources available, there should be no difficulty in establishing a two way system of communication so that all personnel co-operate to meet the patient's needs.

There are ethical considerations to be observed in respect of treating other doctor's patients other than in an emergency. If, for any reason, it appeared necessary to treat an employee routinely, this should only be undertaken at the written request of that worker's own general practitioner. When referring a worker to any external agency such as a hospital or clinic, a clear written communication should be sent which leaves the recipient in no doubt as to the reason why the matter has been referred, what advice and treatment, if any, has been given and any other relevant information. Failure to communicate clearly and at the right time could constitute professional negligence and may have unfortunate repercussions for both occupational health nurse and patient. The relationship between the occupational health nurse and doctor at the place of work has a special significance, and will now be discussed.

Nurse-Doctor Relationship

The traditional roles of both doctor and nurse are changing rapidly due to technological advancement and the perceived priorities of both professions. The Florence Nightingale Pledge for nurses, prepared in 1893,[3] states:

With loyalty will I endeavour to aid the physician in his work and devote myself to the welfare of those committed to my care.

Today the nursing profession is vested with the responsibility of determining its own development and standards of practice. It is a fundamental responsibility of the nurse to promote health, to prevent illness, to restore health and to alleviate suffering'.[4] The nurse must carry out these responsibilities with skill and competence and in a manner consistent with national laws.

The traditional doctor and nurse relationship is founded upon the care of the sick and injured in hospital. In this setting, doctors and nurses work closely together. The doctor examines every new patient, makes a differential diagnosis, if necessary with the use of specialist resources, and prescribes a treatment. The nurses carry out the prescribed treatment, plan and give nursing care. A doctor is often resident and on call day and night to deal with any change in a patient's condition reported by the nursing staff.

By contrast, in an occupational health setting, the nurse invariably plays a different role in acting as point of first contact when the worker reports sickness or illness and it is for the nurse to decide what course of action to adopt. Most patients are examined and treated by occupational health nurses without having been seen by a doctor.

The availability of doctors to support the occupational health nursing services is very variable, ranging from full-time career doctors qualified in occupational health to general practitioners retained to provide clinical support on a sessional basis. Some nurses may have as little as one hour per week of privately arranged doctor time and many others will have none.

No occupational health nurse is ever completely isolated from doctors even if her employer has not made any private arrangements with one. If a patient's condition concerns the nurse, she is always able to contact the employee's general practitioner or the nearest hospital Accident and Emergency Department. If the nurse is concerned because of an occupational cause, the advice of the Employment Medical Advisory Service with their specialist support services is always available and should be used.

The nurse has an important role to play as a practitioner of first contact and must be able to exercise professional skills in order to make an accurate diagnosis of the condition presented and decide the action to be taken in the best interests of the patient. Once emergency measures have been instituted, the nurse may decide to refer the patient to a doctor for further assessment and treatment.

This approach highlights the important differences between the work of a nurse and doctor in a hospital and in an Occupational Health

Service. There is considerable flexibility locally and the rigid distinction between a medical and a nursing task is unclear. The basis upon which the nurse will deal with a problem or refer to a doctor is dependent upon:

1. The restraints of national laws on the nurse's role.
2. The level of the nurse's professional competence.
3. The local policy in operation to deal with injury or sickness arising at work agreed between the doctors and nurses concerned, with the employer.

In the latter, the need for a joint medical and nursing policy is indicated in those situations where the nurse is able to call upon available medical resources. In the event of no medical resources being available, the nurse would have to contain clinical activity within the first two points.

The General Nursing Council for England and Wales, in response to representations made by the Rcn Society of Occupational Health Nursing issued a statement[5] in March 1978 to guide the occupational health nurse who was carrying out treatment procedures not taught in basic nurse training. This statement should form the basis of a local policy agreement so that the circumstances in which a particular treatment is administered are clearly stated in a document signed by the appropriate doctor and nurse and particular treatments should have been clearly authorised in a document signed by the appropriate doctor, after consultation with the nurse. Any such treatment should only be regarded as 'authorised' if all the doctors in a particular occupational health team are in agreement about the form of treatment. Where ongoing treatment is involved, consultation with the patient's general practitioner is essential. When the required treatment or procedure falls outside the normal role of the trained nurse, the nurse should indicate her willingness and competence to carry it out, preferably by signing a document to this effect.

When the treatment concerned involves a technical procedure not normally embraced within the basic training of the trained nurse, the doctor(s) concerned should have instructed the nurse in the procedure (or become satisfied as to her competence) and provide the nurse with a signed authorisation valid for that work situation. The emphasis here is focused upon the need for the doctor to be satisfied about the competence of the nurse and for authorisation to be for that particular employment only.

It will be noted that neither the nursing nor medical bodies have drawn up a list of medical treatments and nursing treatments because of the rapid advances in practice. After their basic training, nurses should undertake specialised courses to equip them to function in a specialist area of clinical practice, where this is clearly indicated for the nature of the work they are to undertake, e.g. ophthalmic procedures.

The British Medical Association and the Royal College of Nursing have produced a joint statement which offers broad guidance to nurses who are concerned about performing duties which fall outside their basic nurse training. This joint statement emphasises the main principles to be observed before any new procedure is undertaken by a nurse in order to offer protection to the patient, the nurse or doctor and the employer.

The Professional Ethic

The nurse is free to exercise discretion and, apart from certain clinical treatment situations, is able to enjoy a wide degree of autonomy. There are safeguards voluntarily accepted in the exercise of this role embodied in the professional ethic.

The occupational health nurse, in addition to building up a body of knowledge and expertise in nursing, is also building up an attitude of mind in the employee, who is, for most of the time, relating to the nurse as a fit and healthy person and only occasionally, when troubled, ill or injured, as a patient. The occupational health nurse does, however, continue a professional relationship with all employees or workers, whether they are fit and well or patients in need of specific nursing help. This relationship is a constant challenge based on the need for the occupational health nurse to adapt continually to changing circumstances, to refrain from taking sides in disputes, to remain a confidante and friend to all and to provide excellence in all she does.

It should go without saying that an occupational health nurse should respect confidences and protect the interests of the client as well as the employer. It sometimes happens that these interests will conflict. Where this happens, the patient's interests must be protected so that no action should be taken by the nurse which may breach the code of confidentiality which must exist between the individual patient and the nurse.

The exercise of tact and the development of good inter-personal relationships are the hallmarks of the occupational health nurse. In order to be able to do this effectively, the nurse must be able to achieve a degree of detachment from all the client group influences, which imping on her role as described in this chapter.

Notes

1. The Director of Education, Royal College of Nursing of the United Kingdom, Henrietta Place, Cavendish Square, London, W1M OAB, England.
2. Especially *Occupational Health*, Bailliere Tindall, London.
3. The Florence Nightingale Pledge, Farrand Training School Committee of Harper Hospital, Detroit, Special Committee (1893).
4. International Council of Nurses Code for Nurses' Ethical Concepts applied to Nursing (1973).
5. The Investigating Committee of the General Nursing Council for England and Wales (1978).

3 PLANNING, FUNCTION AND LAYOUT OF AN OCCUPATIONAL HEALTH DEPARTMENT

Ivor Swanson

The gradual and steady growth during the last decade of Occupational Health Services in industrial and commercial concerns, construction industries, hospital and travel services has been the result of a number of factors. Greater opportunities and improvements in occupational health training, additional legislation covering health at work, recommendations of various government committees and the availability of new and improved methods of diagnosis and treatment have all added to the demand by management, trade unions and employees for comprehensive occupational health services. In spite of this demand, little thought or guidance has been given to the provision of properly designed and equipped health departments, where full use can be made of medical and nursing skills. Trained staff are too often seen attempting to establish and maintain a health service without essential purpose-designed facilities.

Existing Legislation

At present there is no statutory requirement for employers to provide health departments, other than the 'ambulance rooms' required in certain industries — foundries, chemical and clay works, shipbuilding and construction industries. A full detailed list of these Regulations are given in the Notes at the end of the chapter.

A study of the existing United Kingdom legislation, enforced between 1916 and 1966, reveals that the provisions are usually limited to an 'ambulance room' or 'First Aid station' of a minimum size of 100 square feet and having hot and cold water, a sink, table, couch and stretchers and means of sterilising instruments.

Today, the existing Regulations are out of date and totally inadequate in their recommendations if related to modern occupational medicine and nursing practice. A number of large and medium-sized industrial concerns have provided medical departments, manned by trained staff, albeit of varying qualities and offering differing services, and have had the foresight to realise that the advantages of such a facility are not only to the direct benefit of employees, but have also been a proven factor in reducing rates of absenteeism, maintaining production schedules and minimising labour relations problems. Indeed, many of these employers, by providing such facilities, have indirectly been pioneers in the field of occupational health. If it is accepted that a more uniform national Occupational Health Service is desirable, then new legislation is urgently required to provide employees in all industries, offices, research and laboratory premises, educational establishments and hospitals with a revised standard of health care, facilities and trained staff.

Planning a Health Department

There are many advantages if the department can be located in a new building designed solely for the purpose or as part of a new facility housing other office functions. In many instances, however, it is necessary to accept and adapt an existing portion of the factory building. Whichever alternative is available, it is essential to realise that the successful planning of a Health Department is only achieved through teamwork with other professional disciplines.

The planning group should consist of the architect, building contractor, plant engineer, finance staff, together with senior medical and nursing representatives.

Planning a new department can be divided into a number of distinct stages, as follows:

(a) Seek preliminary management approval of the availability of capital to finance the project. It is pointless and time wasting to engage expensive expertise to assist in preparing plans if management are unable to release capital investment funds.

(b) Ascertain the management policy towards initiating and maintaining the type of Occupational Health Service required, viz: a treatment service only or a full service with the accent on preventive health measures.

(c) Examine an outline plan (if a new building) or detailed plan (if existing facility is to be adapted), with the Plant Engineer. In either case the plans should include measurements of the area available, position of stanchions (usually immovable), main service runs of electricity, gas, water, drainage, heating and ventilation.

(d) Visit the proposed site and note the following:

(i)   ease of access to main working areas;

(ii)   ease of access to public highways, noting any specific traffic bottlenecks, e.g. level crossings;

(iii)   the location of outside services – hospitals and

ambulance stations;

(iv)   the number of employees and shift patterns. Note any special groups, e.g. apprentices or employees engaged on high risk jobs;

(v)   the type of manufacture and its hazards;

(vi)   the necessity to be in close proximity to safety, personnel, employment and fire departments;

(vii)   ensure the department is situated on ground level and away from excessively dusty and noisy operations.

(e) Prepare a preliminary internal layout plan together with written details of the size, purpose, services and building finishes required for each room for presentation to architect, contractor and plant engineer for comment, revision and approval.

(f) Prepare a written project including justification for the facility and details mentioned in (d) above and present to the Plant Engineer and finance staff for the addition of detailed costing figures.

(g) Submit a final draft of the project, with costings, details and plans to management for final financial approval.

It is at stage (e) that there should be the greatest involvement of medical and nursing staff. The positioning of rooms within the outline plan, the services, finishes and building furniture should, in the main, be their choice. It is only the department staff who understand work flows and patterns and therefore the grouping of rooms with related work functions should be their decision. Work functions — those of patient care — require certain basic equipment positioned within a room in order to achieve maximum utility with minimum effort and it is the selection and grouping of the equipment and furniture that principally decides the room size. To the staff, the department is a working environment and therefore should be light, comfortable, pleasantly decorated and supplied with functional equipment to reduce effort and time wastage. Finally, before attempting to allocate room positions within the outline plan it is essential to remember the following:

— the type of service offered: viz. treatment or full occupational health facility;
— adaptability: the department must have sufficient space for first aid treatment in the event of a major accident. Some visiting services, such as optician and chiropodist, could utilise one room. Record and store areas must be capable of expansion.

Internal Layout

Rooms and areas fall into one of three service categories.

A. *Treatment* – includes the principal treatment area, showers, resuscitation/casualty rooms, eye treatment, rest rooms, physiotherapy, dental, chiropody, optician, ambulance bay or garage.

B. *Preventive* – comprises consulting rooms, changing cubicles, pre-placement examination area, pathological and industrial hygiene laboratories.

C. *Ancillary* – embraces waiting rooms, toilets, secretarial and record rooms, stores, staff rooms, lecture/library/conference room and all corridor areas. An X-ray department with its supportive services of dark room and film filing area serves both treatment and preventive services.

From experience, the retention of rooms in their three broad categories within the outline plan, usually offers the most practical use of the total area available. The most frequently used rooms, treatment, rest rooms, consulting and secretarial areas, should be allotted sources of natural light. Unnecessary corridors are wasteful of space, but should be of sufficient width in treatment areas to allow ease of stretcher access. Where possible, internal walls should be kept in straight runs – avoid bends, they waste space and money. Similarly, wash basins, showers and toilets should be retained in straight runs throughout the department and if possible located on outside walls, reducing lengthy and costly drainage systems. If sealed inspection traps to the drains are required within the department, it is wise to request their siting away from frequently used treatment rooms, where any overflow will not disrupt service.

Practical Planning

The task of allocating individual rooms within the total area is time consuming, but careful thought at this stage prevents miscalculations and omissions resulting in an ill-designed facility. Once built, it is often impossible, or at best very costly, to redesign a room or readjust the placing of furniture and equipment into an improved layout.

It is wise not to commence drawing the position of rooms and areas on the outline plan, as frequent revision of thought involves the planner in much erasing and redrawing. Place the outline plan to one side and draw each room on a separate piece of squared paper, using the same scale. Each room plan should show the position of doors, windows, furniture, equipment, sanitary ware and necessary services.

The planner should give thought to the work functions to be performed within the room, going through each function or procedure, step by step, listing the equipment required and the needs of the patient and staff, to successfully fulfil that function. To this is added the necessary working space surrounding the equipment.

With large treatment and pre-placement examination areas it is beneficial to sketch in a 'tread plan' or 'flow chart' showing the main walking directions of patients and staff undertaking treatments and examinations. In this manner the distances between waiting areas and treatment or examination rooms, treatment and storage units, treatment/examination and recording area/exit are reduced to a minimum and often decide the optimum position of items of equipment and stores.

With the completion of a plan for each room, the planner should trim the pieces of paper to the edges of the room and finally arrange them within the outline plan of the whole department.

Construction, Finishes and Services

The following notes constitute a basic working knowledge of the various building requirements, services and finishes that are available and allow easier discussion with engineering and construction experts.

(a) Walls. External walls should be at least 11 inch brick, cavity constructed and insulated, with an internal rendering of plaster and finished with several coats of good quality matt or silk emulsion paint or tiled. External rendering will, in most instances, conform to the general appearance and style of the surrounding factory buildings. Internal painted walls can be washed frequently and have the advantage that a colour scheme can be changed at a later date. Tiled surfaces are also easily washed, but with the passing of time, the grouting between the tiles becomes stained and needs to be raked out and re-applied. Compared with tiled walls, a single colour painted surface gives a greater sense of space — an important feature to be considered in a small department.

Internal walls may be 4½ inch single brick, breeze or building block, plastered and painted and should be used where maximum privacy is required, as for consulting rooms. Alternatives can be metal or metal and opaque glass partitioning; being movable they have the advantage of allowing alteration in internal room arrangements. Recent years have seen the increased use of laminated plastic wall sheeting both as an internal finish to walls and as partitioning. This material is free from maintenance problems, other than washing, and can be utilised as splash-backs to wash basins, sinks and laboratory benches.

Black vinyl skirting strips can be utilised in all rooms, with the advantages of rounding the wall and floor union, thus avoiding dirt trapping corners and as a protection to walls from cleaning machines.

Walls, floors and ceilings to X-ray rooms must be constructed to ensure that radiation does not penetrate into adjacent rooms and the use of barium plaster or lead sheet may be necessary. It is advisable to seek the advice of the National Radiological Protection Board at the design stage of X-ray facilities. The Board can also carry out a survey on completion to ascertain that the design requirements have been met. Advice on warning signs, protection for the radiographer and monitoring of exposure is also available.

(b) Floors. Probably the most practical flooring materials to be considered for the majority of rooms are heavy duty industrial vinyl tiles or sheeting laid on a concrete base. They are produced in a variety of patterns and colours, are resilient to wear and easily maintained provided they are correctly washed and sealed. Heavy quality linoleum is also suitable, but compared with vinyl is unlikely to give the same years of service. Terrazzo flooring is extremely hard wearing and washable, but should be used only in selected areas, such as resuscitation, casualty receiving and minor operations rooms, because of its expense. It can be used impressively as a decorative feature in entrance halls.

(c) Ceilings. These may be constructed of plaster board, skim finished and painted. An alternative is to consider ceiling tiles, again painted to the required colour, but it is as well to remember their fire risk. A height of 10 feet from floor to ceiling is adequate — anything greater tends to be wasteful of heat and space.

(d) Windows. Framing may be in wood or metal, the latter being easier to maintain. The opening lights can be hinged outwards or sliding. Where finance allows, double glazing gives the added advantages of reducing noise and heat loss and admits less dust.

(e) Doors. All doors should have a minimum width of 3 feet to allow

ease of stretcher access. Preferably a door should be set in the corner of a room and hinged to open against a wall, thus saving precious space and allowing greater mobility for room equipment. Door construction should be plain, omitting dust catching ledges and panels. Furniture may include safe release locks, door stays, finger and kick plates. Main entrance and exit doors are often doubled to eliminate draughts and heat loss caused by constant use. The distance between two sets of doors should be at least stretcher length to allow easy handling of the patient. The wall space between the doors may be used for directional notices, information boards and health and safety promotion material. Automatic opening entrance doors, governed by a photo-electric cell, are a beneficial luxury. Doors to X-ray rooms must be lead-lined.

(f) Lighting. Natural lighting is essential in any room where treatment is undertaken and in offices and consulting rooms in constant use by staff and patients. In addition, artificial lighting to give an illumination level of at least 800 lux is essential. Probably the best source of electric light is from fluorescent tubes, enclosed and recessed into the ceiling. Lower illumination levels for toilets, store rooms and changing cubicles are acceptable.

Additional local illumination may be necessary in treatment areas, resuscitation and casualty rooms. It is advisable to avoid wide variation of general lighting between adjacent areas.

Much useful information related to illumination levels, light sources and the design and spacing of fittings is available from the Electricity Council and The Illuminating Engineering Society.

Battery operated emergency lighting for corridors, treatment areas and casualty rooms should also be provided. A Code of Practice covering all aspects of emergency lighting is available from the British Standards Institute, B.S. no. 5266.

(g) Heating. Where possible utilise the factory heating system — it may be hot air intake combined with extraction to maintain a warm, constantly filtered and changed atmosphere, or it could be a hot water radiator system. Whatever the system, a temperature of 70°F is comfortable for both patients and staff. Wall thermometers should be placed in areas of constant use.

A source of quick heat, such as electric fan heaters, would provide emergency heating should the main system fail; however, it is wise to remember that these should not be used in rooms where inflammable vapours such as ether, are used. During extremely hot weather these fans may be used as additional cold air blowers.

(h) Ventilation. Open windows provide the easiest form of ventilation, but the disadvantages of noise, dust and smells will almost certainly require the installation of some form of mechanical ventilation, preferably with a filter system to reduce the intake of dirt. If a combined heating and ventilating system is installed factory wide, the department will be well served. Failing this, consider wall and window intake/extract fans. A minimum ventilation rate may be required for medical examination areas and changing cubicles. Advice and information on both ventilation and heating are available from The Chartered Institute of Building Services.

(i) Water Supply, Drainage and Sanitary Fittings. Piped supplies of running hot, cold and drinking water are essential. Where there is a difficulty in supplying hot water, e.g. on a building construction site, a small electric storage water heater can be installed. If drinking water is piped separately to cold supplies, it should be clearly labelled. Separate toilet accommodation should be provided for both patients and staff. Washbasins should always be installed in toilet areas. If space is at a premium there is a choice of corner or recessed models to consider. The choice of sanitary fittings of all types is wide and the most expensive is not necessarily the best value; therefore seek the advice of the building contractor, plant engineer, or visit a Building Centre Information Department. Facilities for showering may be a necessity where the production processes require the use of chemicals and corrosive substances. Again, there is a wide choice of shower units, some portable, with quick, easy installation. Fittings are available in a wide and sometimes bewildering variety of sizes, shapes and finishes. Generally, they are a matter of personal selection, but two items are worthy of consideration: first, swivel mixer tap units with conventional or elbow operated handles, and secondly, toilet odour extract systems which operate with the flushing mechanism. Finally, all water supply and drainage pipes should be concealed within the wall construction.

(j) Electricity. It is not necessary to discuss wiring diagrams and voltages with the electrical installation contractor. However, it is essential to supply him with a list of all electrical equipment to be used in each room together with an exact location of required socket outlets. Details of requirements should include single or multiple sockets, switched or non-switched, bench or wall mounted, and if the latter, the

exact location of installation including height from floor level. A useful check list includes heaters, fans, clocks, infra red lamps, refrigerator, kettles, cooker, eye and inspection magnifying lamps, desk lamps, electrocardiograph, vitalograph, audiometry apparatus and booths, cleaning machines, outside power socket for ambulance heater connection, X-ray viewing screens, patient call systems and internal security alarms. Special arrangements may be required for cabling and wiring circuits if the department is to include X-ray, physiotherapy or dental services. These services call for consultation between the electrical contractor and the manufacturers of the selected equipment.

(k) Telephones. Even in the smallest department, two telephone lines are essential, both situated in the main treatment area. Line one, for incoming internal emergency calls only, should be connected to a receiving instrument without a dialling-out facility, but with switched extension to first aid room or security office in order that emergency calls are answered when the medical department is unmanned. Line two should have normal internal and external dialling systems and extensions from this line to the medical officer's room should be considered. In larger departments, additional lines may be necessary to X-ray, staff rooms, and pre-placement examination areas.

(l) Fire Precautions. A suitable number and type of fire extinguishers should be provided to fight both conventional and electrical fires. Their siting would include main entrances, treatment area, X-ray, physiotherapy and staff rooms. Large departments may be included in any factory-wide smoke detection and automatic sprinkler systems and may include a fire location indicator board and bell alarm. Fire exit notices should be placed in all corridors. Advice on fire precaution problems can always be sought from the factory fire officer or the local brigade's fire prevention officer. Staff should be taught the precaution of storing bottled inflammable liquids in a metal container situated in a cool area away from any source of heat. Similarly, oxygen and gas cylinders require storage in a cool area. The areas of both hazards should display NO SMOKING or NAKED LIGHTS notices.

Colour Schemes

As mentioned elsewhere, the department is the working environment of the staff and, therefore, a pleasantly decorated area does much to maintain morale and job satisfaction. Above all, a cold, austere clinical appearance should be avoided. A great deal of advice on the merits of various colour schemes is available from literature and building and decorating agencies. However, it is worth recording a few basic guide lines.

Colours can be divided into 'fixed' and 'changeable' colours.

Fixed colours — those of plastic laminates, wall and floor tiles, blankets and vinyl coverings to furniture. These are items that will be part of the room for a considerable number of years and for the first three materials it is probably wise to choose white, cream, grey or buff shades. Mottled or striped patterns should be used for laminates and floor tiles to avoid scratch marks showing. Plain colours can be employed for wall tiles. Strong, definite colours can be used in the choice of blankets and vinyl materials.

Changeable colours — those of paint for walls, ceilings, doors, window frames, curtaining and screening materials, as they can be altered more frequently. The most practical changeable colours for walls are ivory, cream and pastel shades which give a sense of space to a limited area. The only exception is the colour of eye treatment room walls, which are generally finished in matt black paint to give the greatest possible background contrast for ophthalmic spotlight illumination. Stronger colours can be used on doors, windows, framing and in curtaining, either as a complete contrast to or as a deeper shade of a paler wall colour. Ceilings are invariably finished in a white non-reflecting paint.

In planning colour schemes, it is not only the colours of the walls, woodwork, floors and ceilings that require co-ordination; the shades of furnishing fabrics, tiles, laminates, screening and curtaining materials and blankets should all be included in the total appearance of the facility. The planner is advised to obtain colour samples of all materials to be employed within the department and to spend time matching shades into a total co-ordinated scheme. Samples should include swatches of upholstery, curtaining and laminates, while paint colours should be selected from the British Standards Institute's 'Paint Colours for Building Purposes', B.S.4800:1972.

Requests to the building contractor for colour choices for wall and woodwork paint finishes should be made from this list, quoting the B.S. number. Listed in Table 3.1 are a number of suggested colour schemes, all of which have been employed in recent departmental designs, for those who find the problem difficult and the choice bewildering.

Table 3.1: Suggested Colour Schemes

Item	Scheme 1	Scheme 2	Scheme 3	Scheme 4	Scheme 5	Scheme 6
Walls	Ivory 10 B.15	Ivory 10 B.15	Mushroom Pink 04 C 33	Ivory 10 B.15	Narvic Blue 18 E 49	Vanilla 08 C 31
Woodwork	Light Grey 10 A 03	Olive Green 12 D 45	Chestnut Brown 06 C 39	Chestnut Brown 06 C 39	Smoke Blue 18 D 43	Chestnut Brown 06 C 39
Floor Tiles	Grey/White streaked	Buff/White Grey/White streaked	Grey/White streaked	Buff/White streaked 1	Grey/White Buff/White streaked	Buff/White streaked
Vinyl or Fabric Furniture covering	Pimento Orange or Chestnut Brown	Purple	Cornflower Blue	Palm Green	Chestnut Brown	Palm Green or Tangerine
Blankets	White	Light Green	White	Light Green	Cream	Green or White
Curtaining or Screening	White or Ivory	White background, bold flower/leaf pattern in Purple and Greens.	White or Ivory	White background, bold leaf/grass pattern in Browns and Black.	White background, bold flower/leaf pattern in Blues, Browns and Black	White or Ivory

Furniture and Equipment

The quantity and variety of equipment necessary for each occupational health department will vary according to the size and hazards of the industry concerned, the number of employees and the variety of treatments and examinations undertaken. The notes below are intended to give an awareness of the range of equipment manufactured and to leave the final choice to the reader.

(a) Office Furniture, Chairs and Couches

These requirements constitute the largest number of items in any department. Office furniture, including desks, filing cabinets, stationery and storage cabinets, tables and chairs, should be purchased from one manufacturer to ensure a continuity of style, shape and colour throughout the department. Several manufacturers now supply examination couches, foot stools, arm and leg rests, styled and upholstered in matching vinyl or fabric materials to those utilised on chairs.

Desks are manufactured in wood or steel framing with or without pedestal drawer units, with wood or laminate tops — the latter probably being more hardwearing and practical to clean.

Chairs with wood or stove enamelled, chrome or nylon coated steel frames come in a wide variety of styles: static or swivel, with or without arms, upholstered in vinyl or fabric material in a wide range of colours. Vinyl coverings are especially suitable in areas of heavy use or where likely to be contaminated with oil or dirt. Easy cleaning, using soapy water and a soft brush, is an added advantage. Stacking chairs are worthy of consideration in rooms that have a dual role — for example, a waiting area that can be cleared for use as a First Aid training room or a physiotherapy unit that occasionally doubles as a lecture room.

Upholstered bench units with integrated tables can be an attractive feature of a waiting room.

Couches — the frame can be wood or stove enamelled, chrome or nylon coated steel, while the upholstery is nearly always vinyl.

An adjustable head end with a secure fixing device is essential. Varieties include extra low couches for certain physiotherapy treatments, extra wide model for ECG examinations, recessed head end legs to allow staff to sit comfortably at eye treatments.

Accessories to couches include clip-on padded arm rests, brackets for intravenous infusion bottles and inspection lamps, and rollers and troughs for disposable paper sheeting.

Stationery and Filing Cabinets — both items should be purchased with locks. The former, which can be obtained with additional shelves if required, are excellent as relatively cheap storage units for most types of medical stores. A recent addition to the market has been the introduction of a basic stationery cabinet fitted with varying sized plastic boxes enabling even the smallest items such as eye and skin medicaments and injection materials to be stored neatly.

(b) Medical Furniture

Dressing and Treatment Trolleys are manufactured in stove enamelled, chrome or nylon coated steel with glass or metal shelves. The most popular sizes are 18″ x 18″ or 24″ x 18″ and can be supplied with or without guard rails and drawer units. The addition of the latter feature almost doubles the cost. Anti-static castors are essential.

Instrument Cabinets with glass fronted doors, once popular items of equipment with serried ranks of instruments on display, are now displaced by sterile pack dispensers, more useful and cheaper articles of furniture.

Paper Towel Holders, Waste Bins and Sack Holders — paper towelling has been a feature of modern medical units for a considerable number of years now and has contributed greatly towards reducing the risk of cross infection. Planners should initially decide the type of paper towel required as opposed to the towel holder. Factors, in order of importance, include absorbency, size, texture and presentation, i.e. interleaved or perforated roll.

Waste bins consist of a metal bin with a foot operated lid and accommodate an internal paper or polythene liner. They can be wall mounted or free standing; most are fire retardant and many are finished in epoxy powder coating in a variety of colours.

Sack holders are simpler, consisting of a circular head unit over which a paper or polythene sack is folded and held in position with a clamping ring. The head can be wall mounted or fitted to a floor standing frame with foot operated lid.

Waste bins are probably more acceptable to a medical unit if stability, appearance and fire resistance are more important.

Working Bench and Dressings Units — the time honoured method of practising patient treatment from a dressing trolley appears in recent years to have become less popular in both technique and layout. The recently favoured method of working from a fixed bench unit which incorporates sink units, storage facilities, waste disposal, drug cupboard and pack dispenser reduces the nurse's 'tread pattern' to a minimum, saving time and effort for both patient and staff. These comprehensive units were originally designed to be fixed against a wall, but similarly constructed smaller units may be used back to back in multiples of two, three or four units to form 'island' treatment centres in large occupational health departments.

Several manufacturers offer a very wide variety of bench, cupboard, drawer and sink modules designed to be used singly or grouped in arrangements to meet varying departmental requirements. Features of these modules include melamine finishes to all internal and external surfaces, magnetic door catches, recessed handles, choice of internal drawer divisions and doors hinged to give 180° openings.

Personal lockers – each member of staff requires a lockable cupboard of sufficient depth or width to store off duty clothes on hangers and separate shelving to accommodate supplies of clean uniform, duty shoes and personal effects.

Ophthalmic Inspection and Magnifying Lamps – the accurate and successful diagnosis and treatment of eye injuries and conditions depends to a very large extent on the availability of a good quality ophthalmic lamp. The model chosen should have a magnifying lens to give an even spotlight of intense illumination over a small area. Most models are supplied with a transformer, and are available with wall or floor mounting. A magnifying lamp is an extremely useful item of equipment in departments where the removal of splinters and other close, accurate treatment procedures are frequently undertaken. Probably the most practical instrument manufactured for this purpose consists of a magnifying head and lens, using a 22 watt circular fluorescent tube, mounted on balanced arms allowing the magnifier to be placed in any fixed position, leaving the operator's hands free for treatment purposes. A 3 diopter lens is fitted as standard, but additional clip on lenses, 7 or 11 diopter power, can be obtained. The cool fluorescent tube allows close work without discomfort to the patient, while wall, bench or floor standing trolley gives a choice of mounting.

Wheelchairs – a study of manufacturers' catalogues reveals a wide range of chair, frame, castor, arm and back styles and sizes. The most useful model for use within the factory environment is a folding adult chair with swivel 8 inch front castors to give ease of steering. The folding feature allows the chair to fit into a car boot, an important consideration if the patient is to be transported to hospital or home.

Folding ambulance chairs of the type utilised by most county ambulance services are useful in transporting patients through narrow aisleways and twisting stairways. Variations in design include 2 or 4 wheel models, with or without footrest and extra wide safety straps.

Stretchers — simple *standard* stretchers consisting of lightweight metal poles, rigid or folding, with canvas or nylon coated plastic carrying sheets are essential items of equipment in any industrial concern. Additional sets of poles and sheets are useful and cheap items of emergency equipment for major accident incidents.

Trolley stretchers manufactured with a light alloy metal framework, fitted with anti-static castors and canvas or metal bed tops are used extensively for the conveyance of patients from the factory workshop to the medical department. The smallest recommended castors to negotiate varying floor levels are 8 inches in diameter. At least two of the four wheels should be supplied with foot operated brakes, preferably at diagonally opposite corners. Accessories include equipment tray, intravenous transfusion stand, oxygen cylinder rack and restraint and retaining straps. Other more sophisticated models have the ability to adjust to a reclining chair stretcher, while ambulance trolley stretchers capable of varying height adjustment are available from many manufacturers.

Rescue stretchers — in industries where special problems of casualty rescue have been encountered (from high buildings, underground tanks, places of awkward or limited access) the 'Neil Robertson' has been the stretcher of choice. However, over the past decade, the 'Paraguard' stretcher has become an increasingly popular item of rescue equipment. This stretcher is built on two durable lightweight metal poles between which are foam cushions. Security of the patient is maintained by restraining harnesses and straps fastened by quick release adjustable buckles. The framing poles are detachably jointed allowing the patient to be transported around difficult corners and tight spaces. Accessories include a four-point lifting sling, lowering line and guide ropes, slot-in carrying handles and shoulder harness.

Scoop stretchers are worthy of mention, being of all-metal construction with an automatic end latch hinge allowing the stretcher to open in its length. The patient is 'scooped' into the stretcher by a scissor action and this item is ideal for difficult pick ups with minimal discomfort and disturbance to the victim.

Oxygen and Resuscitation Apparatus — the marketed range of oxygen giving apparatus is wide and offers the occupational health nurse a choice of options from the simple portable inhalers to sophisticated automatic resuscitators, giving positive-negative pressure, complete with suction unit. Factors that should influence the purchase of such equipment would include portability, weight, length of operation, simplicity of use, oxygen concentrations required and the availability of a quick, reliable maintenance service.

Suction Equipment — a clear airway is a necessity prior to resuscitation. Indeed, a simple suction unit is of more value than oxygen apparatus — for once an airway is established, resuscitation can be effectively accomplished by 'mouth to mouth' breathing and external cardiac massage. At least two small, simple and effective suction units are now available that do not require electric power for operation. The first consists of a container with inlet and outlet ports, catheter connection and hand bulb. Suction is achieved by creating a vacuum by depressing the bulb. It could be used by trained non-medical staff. The second is composed of a vacuum bottle to which a suction unit of a pressurised disposable cartridge containing a non-toxic, non-inflammable gas is fitted. The unit is hung around the neck of the operator, leaving the hands free to direct the catheter which is attached to the vacuum bottle. Operation is by turning a knurled knob and can be maintained, if necessary continuously, for 20 to 30 minutes.

Analgesic Apparatus — the relatively recent acceptance of a mixture of 50 per cent nitrous oxide, 50 per cent oxygen as an analgesic beneficial to patients with severe injury, coronary distress and other painful medical conditions has been of considerable aid to nursing staff. The mixture can be self-administered by the patient and is often a preferred alternative to drugs of opiate derivation. The relief of pain usually begins after 20 seconds of inhalation and is maximal after 1½ minutes. There are no after effects, no masking of symptoms and it is compatible with other drugs. It can be administered by trained nursing staff without medical supervision.

Notes

Existing Legislation requiring 'Ambulance Rooms' or 'First Aid Stations'

Blast Furnaces, Copper Mills, Iron Mills, Foundries and Metal Works, S.R. & O. 1917, no. 1067.
Saw Mills and Woodworking Factories, S.R. & O. 1918, no. 1489.
Oil Cake Manufacture, S.R. & O. 1929, no. 534.
Chemical Works, S.R. & O. 1922, no. 731.
Herring Curing, S.R. & O. 1926, no. 535; 1927, no. 813.
Clay Works, S.I. 1948, no. 1547.
Shipbuilding & Ship Repairing, S.I. 1960, no. 1932.
Construction, S.I. 1966, no. 95.

Useful Addresses in the UK for Sources of Further Information

The Electricity Council, 30 Millbank, London, SW1P 4RD.

The Illuminating Engineering Society, York House, 199 Westminster Bridge Road, London, SE1 7UN.

The Building Centre, 26 Store Street, London, WC1.

The Design Centre, 28 Haymarket, London, SW1.

The British Hospital Equipment Display Centre, 22 Newman Street, London, W1.

The British Standards Institute, 2 Park Street, London, W1.

The National Radiological Protection Board, Harwell, Didcot, Oxon, OX11 ORQ.

The Chartered Institution of Building Services, 49 Cadogan Square, London, SW1X OJB.

4 RECORDS

Eileen Astbury

Record keeping is an essential and integral part of the occupational health nurse's role. Recording forms a part of other skills and duties in her daily work. It is perhaps not the most interesting or immediately rewarding part of her work, but its importance should not be underestimated.

Records are kept within an occupational health department for many reasons. They have, however, one basic purpose in common: they are kept so that information may be referred to at a later date.

Records fall into two main categories:

1. Statutory, the ones which must be kept by law.
2. Voluntary, those records kept because it is known to be advantageous to do so.

Statutory Records

The records which have to be kept by law will depend on the type of establishment, e.g. factory, mine, hospital, etc., and whether or not there are certain specific hazards to be found there. The occupational health nurse may or may not be responsible for the keeping of the statutory records. She should, however, know about these records and be conversant with their function.

The Factories Act 1961 is one of the most important pieces of legislation to occupational health nurses in Britain. Not only factories are covered by this legislation, but parts of other establishments such as mines and hospitals are also affected.

A. Records required by the Factories Act 1961

(i) The General Register for Factories – F31 HMSO. The factory occupier is responsible for maintaining this register, although the nurse may be asked to keep it within the health department. There are seven parts to the register:

1. General. – the name of the occupier, postal address and type of work carried on are stated. Certificate as to means of escape from fire should be attached to it.

2. Young Persons – under this heading are entered details of the

53

young persons under eighteen taken into employment: names, addresses, date of notice to Careers Office and which Careers Office was informed of their employment.

3. Accidents and Dangerous Occurrences — this part is for the recording of accidents causing loss of life or disabling a worker for more than three days preventing him from earning full wages, and certain listed dangerous occurrences, whether any injury is sustained or not. Details are to be given as to time and date, name of person injured and the precise occupation at time of accident, and how the accident happened. H.M. Factory Inspectorate must be informed by means of Form F43. These forms are at the end of the register, but can be obtained separately. It may be the duty of the occupational health nurse to fill in this form.

4. Cases of Poisoning or Disease — the occupier must enter in this part of the register every case of beryllium, cadmium, lead, phosphorus, manganese, arsenical, mercurial, carbon bisulphide, aniline or chronic benzene poisoning or cases of compressed air illness, toxic jaundice, toxic anaemia, anthrax, epitheliomatous ulceration or chrome ulceration occurring in the factory. Notification is made (a) to the District Inspector of Factories and (b) to the Employment Medical Adviser of the area in which the factory is situated by Form F41 or an interim letter if there is delay in receiving the form. It may be the duty of the occupational health nurse to fill in this document. All cases of this type of poisoning or disease must be notified, even if the worker is not disabled for three days.

5. Washing, painting, whitewashing, etc., of walls — all dates, parts of the factory, type of treatment and who carried out the work are recorded in this part.

6. Testing or examination of fire warning systems — information is required regarding the type of system, the date of the test, any defects found and any action to remedy defects. There are special conditions with regard to the number of workers, date of construction and where there is storage of explosive or flammable material.

7. Persons trained in First Aid — where more than fifty people are employed a First Aid box must be placed in the charge of a person trained in First Aid. The names of the First Aiders, qualifications, date of certificate and inspection of certificate are recorded. The names of State Registered and State Enrolled Nurses should also be included.

Parts 2, 3, 5 and 6 of this Register are also issued as separate books. The register is dated on the front cover, and must be kept available for inspection by H.M. Inspector of Factories and Employment Medical

Advisers, for two years, or other prescribed period, after the date of the last entry.

The overall purpose of this statutory record is for identification of areas of hazard. The information collected through the Health and Safety Executive gives a picture of industrial injury and disease. It pinpoints particular hazards and is designed for control and prevention.

(ii) Health Registers. A statutory record is required to be kept for employees working in certain hazardous processes. This record is used for preventive purposes to ensure that legislation is working properly.

Statutory Instruments lay down the different types of examinations needed for various hazards. A Health Register may be a group register or a personal register, and the records must be kept for various periods for different hazards.

To give examples: *Health Register F 2145 HMSO:* this covers nine different regulations concerned with lead. It is a group Health Register and will take entries for forty-eight employees. Details of the employees and their employment are entered together with the process. There is a section to be completed by the Employment Medical Adviser or the appointed doctor, with particulars of the examination, together with the date and result. The doctor signs a special section if the employee would be at risk to his health if he continued with the process. Within seven days after the end of a calendar month in which the doctor has made the entry, the page containing the carbon copy is removed and sent to H.M. Factory Inspectorate. There is no specified period for this register to be kept.

Register for use with the Chromium Plating Regulations 1931 and 1973 F 2418: the factory occupier arranges for a responsible person (this could be the nurse) to enter the results of the twice-weekly inspection of workers in the Register. This is a group record with a space for the list of the workers' names, and the process, together with the dates of examination. The record must be kept available for inspection for two years (or other prescribed period) after the date of the last entry. A register must also be kept under Chromium Plating Regulations, Regulation 1(a) F 2419, where entries are made of statutory atmospheric monitoring carried out every two weeks.

The Health Register F 2067 HMSO: this is kept under the Ionising Radiations (Sealed Sources) Regulations 1969 and Ionising Radiations (Unsealed Radioactive Substances) Regulations 1968. It is a personal record prepared so that pages can be filed in alphabetical order in a loose leaf binder. This record contains columns for the type of

Table 4.1: Factories Act 1961 — Extract from Health and Safety
Executive Publications Catalogue (HMSO)

Health Registers	Form No.
Carcinogenic Substances (Regulations 1967), Register of Persons subject to medical examination	F 2282
Chemical Works Regulations (Reg. 30(a)) 1972	F 605
Chromium Plating Regulations (Reg. 10)	F 2418
Chromium Plating Regulations (Reg. 1(a))	F 2419
Compressed Air Health Register (Regs. 14 and 15) 1972	F 751
Divers' Fitness Register (Reg. 9) 1972	F 2015
Electric Accumulator Regulations (Reg. 13(b))	F 2145
Heading of Yarn Regulations (Reg. 3)	F 2145
Indiarubber Regulations (Reg. 13(b)) (any fume process) 1972	F 605
Indiarubber Regulations (Reg. 12(b)) (any lead process)	F 2145
Ionising Radiations (URS) Regulations (Reg. 34(1))	F 2067
Ionising Radiations (Sealed Sources) Regulations (Reg. 31(1))	F 2067
Lead Compounds Regulations (Reg. 11(c))	F 2145
Lead Compounds — portable register for Women and Young Persons (Ss. 75 and 128) 1972	F 616
Lead Paint — Register of Persons employed in Painting Buildings and the work on which they are employed (S. 129(4))	F 92
Lead Smelting Regulations (Reg. 13(b))	F 2145
Mule Spinning Regulations (Reg. 6(2)) 1972	F 659
Paints and Colours (Manufacture) Regulations (Reg. 6)	F 2145
Patent Fuel Manufacture Regulations (Reg. 16(4)) 1972	F 625
Pottery Regulations (Reg. 8(1)) (Processes under Reg. 7(1)) 1972	F 2145
Pottery Regulations (Reg. 8(1)) (Processes under Regs. 6(7) and 25) 1972	F 655
Tinning Regulations (Reg. 5)	F 2145
Vitreous Enamelling Regulations (Reg. 8)	F 2145

examination and a section as to fitness. The record is signed by the
Employment Medical Adviser or the appointed doctor, and must be
kept for thirty years after the last entry. A radiation dose record is also
kept. When an employee leaves his employment he is given a transfer
record of his radiation exposure.

The occupational health nurse must be aware of the statutory
records which need to be kept in her organisation. Where she is in doubt
about a process the Employment Medical Advisory Service will advise.

(iii) Codes of Practice. There are requirements under Codes of Practice
for people working with ionising radiations in various establishments
outside the Factories Act 1961. These Codes are designed to
harmonise with factory legislation. Details of these records, which are
also kept for thirty years, are found in the *Code of Practice for the
Protection of Persons Against Ionising Radiations Arising from Medical
and Dental Use,* and *Code of Practice for the Protection of Persons
Exposed to Ionising Radiations in Research and Teaching* (HMSO
Publications).

The Health and Safety Commission are currently looking at the
problems of hazards at the work place. They see the vital need for
improved information for the control and prevention of occupational
ill health and accidents. A series of consultative and draft documents
are being issued, published by HMSO.

In the light of these publications there are likely to be radical
changes in the records required by the Health and Safety Executive.
It is foreseen that the requirements for statutory examinations will
change. There is a growing use of Codes of Practice and Guidance Notes
from the Health and Safety Executive. The occupational health nurse
must be especially vigilant in this time of change, to keep up-to-date
with current practice and information.

B. Records required by the Social Security Act 1975
(Formerly National Insurance (Industrial Injuries) Act 1965.)

Accident Book – Form B1 510 or B1 510 A (the smaller edition). The
Accident Book is kept to benefit the individual employee. This book is
to be placed for use in mines, quarries and factories and other business
premises where ten or more insured people are normally employed at
any one time. It should be kept in a place readily accessible at all
reasonable times to any injured person and any person acting on his
behalf. This book must be provided by the occupier and can be kept
in the health department or in other places in the organisation. It is not
obligatory for the nurse to enter details. The patient himself or
someone acting on his behalf may make the entry. The purpose of the
book is to help an injured person to give notice of his accident to his
employer, as required by regulations under Section 88 of the Social
Security Act 1975.

The details needed are: full name, address and occupation of the
injured person; his signature or that of any other person making the
record, together with their details of address and job; the date of the
entry; time and date of accident; where the accident happened; and

the cause and nature of the injury to the injured person.

The employer is required to investigate the accident and if there is a discrepancy, he has to make a record of this. The Accident Book should be kept for three years from the date of the last entry, and could well be incorporated into the records in the health department, particularly in a small organisation.

Voluntary Records

The types of records kept within any medical department will depend on the type of organisation and the ideas and opinions of the occupational health team. They fall into three main categories.

A. Medical Records.
B. Environmental Records.
C. Administrative Records.

Any system used for these records should be simple to use and to understand. Duplication both of effort and material should be avoided. A record system must always have a purpose; it should be capable of expansion at a later date. Retrieval of information should be as easy as possible.

A. Medical Records

These are kept in the interests of the individual, the organisation concerned, the nurse and the medical officer. It should always be remembered that at some time any information recorded may be needed in a court of law.

Whatever medical records are kept, the same guidelines apply to them all. They should be correct. The information should be accurate as far as is humanly possible. They should be clear. The writing must be legible in a medium which does not blur or fade. The language used should be literate. They should be concise, this enables salient facts to stand out clearly. They should be comprehensive. All the essential facts should be recorded. They should conform to a standard, so that uniformity of records is achieved, for ease of comparison. They must be confidential. The storage and safekeeping of records is an essential part of the work of the department. They should contain all current information available. Out-of-date records may be misleading.

Medical Records generally fall into three main categories:
(i)   the Personal Health Records;
(ii)   the general record of patients attending each day (the 'Day Book');

(iii) records kept for special groups.

Type of documentation. The forms used will depend on the requirements of the medical department and the organisation. Particular care should be taken when starting a new system. Records used by well established firms could be looked at with advantage. Their documents will have been revised over the years and mistakes rectified. It is relatively easy to see flaws in records systems, but difficult to design a new system from the beginning. A pilot scheme may be useful, highlighting the need for amendments, before large-scale printing is undertaken. Forms used should be simple and clear. Standardisation within an organisation makes for ease of working and economy.

Computer facilities are available to an increasing number of medical departments and form design should take into account this modern development. The recommendation to use international A4 size paper in hospital records, made by the Tunbridge Committee in its Report on the Standardisation of Hospital Medical Records in 1965[1] has been followed through in general practice. The 1971 conference of representatives of local medical committees recommended that the future medical record should be of a size to take unfolded paper of A4 size.[2] The advantage of this is that it allows storage of records and reports without the need to fold the documents. This makes for clarity and ease of working. It does, however, take a large amount of storage space. The records kept by a medical department are similar in many ways to those kept in general practice. A4 size notes have been found to work well within the medical services in industry.

It is advantageous if all the documents relating to one person are kept in a suitable envelope, identified on the outside by name only. A coloured envelope may indicate whether it appertains to a male or female employee. Special codes could be used to indicate their department, or if they are working with a particular hazard.

Confidentiality of records. Information contained within the records is confidential. The time taken and materials used to compile the records are paid for by the management, but it is customary and essential to expect this ownership to be waived, so that confidentiality can be maintained. The patient's written permission must be obtained for any disclosure, unless the information is subpoenaed by a court of law.

The problem of confidentiality is a difficult one, but it is still possible for the nurse to be co-operative and helpful without disclosing medical or personal details. Personnel officers and managers need to have certain information when making job placements. They may find nursing ethics hard to understand. However, the nurse can indicate when a job is not suitable, e.g. 'may not climb heights', without discussing a person's disability. To get full use from the Personal Health Record every member of the organisation must be able to trust the confidentiality and safekeeping of their records.

The Safety Representative is entitled to request through the employer to see relevant statutory information but there is no requirement to make non-statutory records available. This is fully discussed in Rcn Information Leaflet no.10.

The storage of records. The safekeeping and method of storage of records needs to be arranged before any records are begun. Expert advice should be obtained to ensure the most suitable system is introduced, e.g. specialist shelving, suspension filing, cabinets, etc. The method chosen will need to take into account the following factors:

(a)   the number of records to be stored – at present and in the future;

(b)   the amount of storage space available;

(c)   funds available.

Whatever system is selected, the security of the records must be ensured. This will entail locking any cabinets, or the room in which the records are stored when unattended. The lock should be of an uncommon type, and its keys available only to the relevant members of the health department team.

Records should be stored logically. This may be alphabetically, in works number order, or a special index may be compiled. Special care needs to be taken when replacing records in the file, to ensure they are in the correct order. Records should not be left lying about the department. It is estimated that within the National Health Service, about 4 per cent of records are misplaced or misfiled.[3] A missing record may be vitally needed. A great deal of embarrassment is caused and time wasted when a record is not in its correct place or not immediately available when required.

The Personal Health Record should be kept as long as it may be needed. The information may have been compiled over many years. The employee may leave the firm; he could well return at a later date. If he transfers to another part of the country within the same firm, in this case, with the employee's consent, his health record could be transferred to the new medical department. A policy on the length of time out-of-date records are stored must be decided within the health department. There should be a written instruction which is understood by all staff dealing with records. It would seem that in view of the long time which can elapse between exposure to a hazard and the development of occupational disease (e.g. occupational deafness, asbestosis, carcinoma of the skin) that records should be kept almost indefinitely. Where many records are involved, the information could be put on microfilm, to ensure safekeeping and to minimise storage space. When the records are eventually disposed of, this should be done by shredding or burning the documents.

Pro-forma letter or record. It could be of great value to the health department to have specially designed forms or letters (e.g. see Figure 4.1). These could incorporate a carbon copy, so that there was the minimum of duplication of work. One type could give information to the safety department with regard to accidents; another could be used for information for a patient's family doctor or hospital. Gentle of the Birmingham Accident Hospital has designed a transfer form for use between hospitals and industrial medical departments.[4] An advantage of this type of record is that the printed information is standardised, and this helps to ensure that vital information is not omitted.

(i) Personal Health Record

The Personal Health Record is a most valuable document. Its use as a guideline enables correct job placement to be made at first employment and if rehabilitation is needed. The initial screening results form a baseline to which to refer at a later date. The patterns of illness and injury in the individual may be followed, indicating the need for other measures. A comprehensive document is built up relating to the health of the individual at work.

The Personal Health Records should include:

(a) Pre-placement or First Health Interview Record.[5] All pre-employment screening findings should be recorded logically and clearly, together with a medical and occupational history. This could be of prime importance if an occupational disease is later found in the employee. Health questionnaires used should be simple to fill in and free from any ambiguity.

The first page should give personal details of the employee: name, address, date of birth, marital status, job, works number, department, date of joining the firm, the name and address of the family doctor, date of any immunisations and vaccinations.

Figure 4.1: Recording of Eye Conditions

An impression made by rubber stamp for use in indicating area of trauma to an eye or location of foreign body.

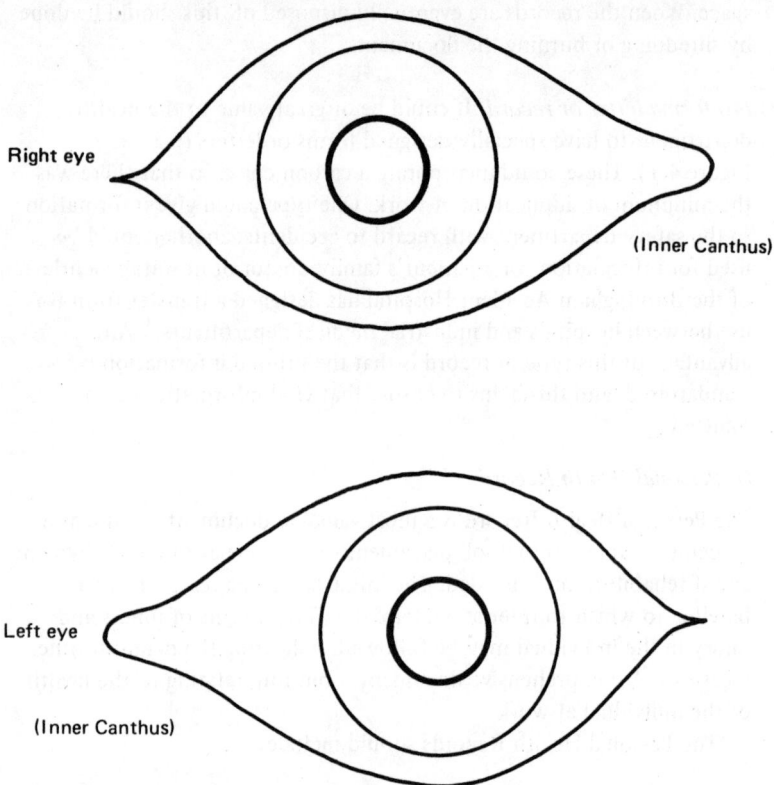

Right eye

(Inner Canthus)

Left eye

(Inner Canthus)

An Eye stamp can be obtained from suppliers of rubber stamps by sending a drawing of the impression needed.

This aid is particularly suitable for use in a letter of referral, a personal health record, or on a treatment card.

Source: British Steel Corporation, Stocksbridge Works, Sheffield.

Arrangements should be made so that all changes in address or job, etc., are up-dated whenever necessary.

A clear panel on the first page could be made:

$$\boxed{\text{Important}}$$

This can be used to give any special or vital details about the employee, e.g. diabetic, any allergy, any special medication, such as steroids. This may be life-saving on occasion.

(b) Individual Health Record. This is the record which contains full details of every attendance by an individual to the occupational health department. Details recorded include: the day and date; the time of arrival in the department; the time of occurrence of any injury or onset of illness; the history of any illness or injury; the record of all screenings or examinations carried out; provisional diagnosis; the treatment or any advice given; details of any referral; the dispersal of the patient — whether he returned to work, went or was taken home or to hospital or referred to a family doctor.

The record should be completed whilst the patient is in the health department. In cases of emergency, details should be entered — even if very briefly — as soon as possible and the record completed as soon as feasible once the emergency is over. The record should be signed by the nurse. Where two nurses have dealt with the patient, both signatures should be entered. On subsequent re-attendances for the treatment of a condition essential information should again be recorded. Any significant developments or referrals should be noted.

Special points in completing the record. The 24-hour clock should be used. Particular care must be taken with the writing of figures, e.g. that a 1 or 2 is not confused with 7. When using the words 'right' or 'left' for the first time in a record, ensure that these words are written out in full.

When identifying fingers the digits must be named: thumb, index, middle, ring and little (see Figure 4.2). It is important that the particular part of the finger affected is named. The aspect should be described, i.e. front (palmar) or back (dorsal).

When identifying toes the digits must again be named: great toe, second, third, fourth and little toe. All descriptions of signs, symptoms or of injury should be as specific as possible. It is not sufficient to say 'swollen ankle', but rather 'swelling over the external malleolus'. When

Figure 4.2: Recording of Hand Conditions

Palmar or front view of left hand

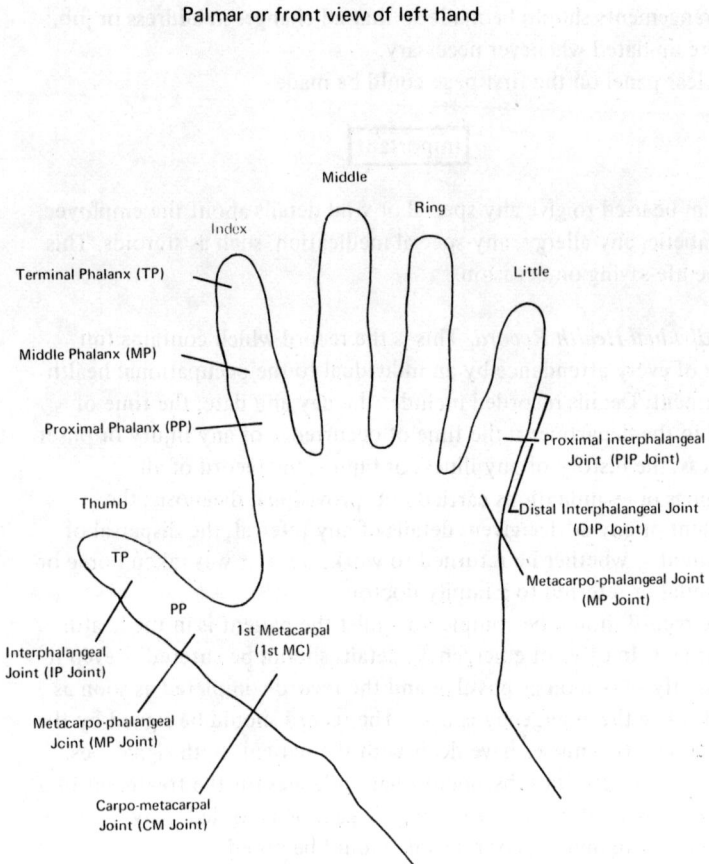

Terminology and acceptable abbreviations for the identification of areas of fingers.

Source: British Steel Corporation, Stocksbridge Works, Sheffield.

describing pain, try to give a picture of the type and location of the pain, e.g. 'griping pain left side of chest radiating down the left arm and into the neck'. Avoid stating that a fracture is present unless this is quite obvious. The identity of any chemical or hazardous substance should be clearly stated if this is known.

With burns the area damaged should be recorded in square centimetres. The depth should be recorded, e.g. reddening of the skin, blistering, blanching of the skin, insensitivity to pain, etc.

Any screening measures must be recorded in full. It is not sufficient to say blood pressure (B.P.) normal, or temperature pulse respiration (T.P.R.) normal. The actual reading should be entered.

Any records indicating the use of Tetanus Toxoid could be underlined in red. It should also be recorded whether it is the first, second or third injection or a booster dose.

Where Controlled Drugs are given it may be useful to have these underlined in red to indicate their use.

Where a patient attends the medical department with a problem he wants to discuss, a record should be made of the attendance with a minimum of detail.

When recording details of an accident, the nurse needs to be concerned as to how the accident occurred and how the patient was injured, and the extent of any trauma. It is not her duty to investigate the accident nor to state her opinion. The phrase 'the patient stated' followed by the patient's account of the accident may prove useful. It is most important that an accurate record of the facts is obtained at this time.

Often a patient is shaken and upset when an accident has occurred and the nurse should avoid trying to take too detailed a statement. The exact situation, the time of the accident and its reporting, the work being done, the cause of the accident and the injury sustained must, however, be recorded. Should any alteration be made to this record, for any reason, the time and date and signature of the person making the alteration must be recorded.

The accident record is particularly important. It establishes the facts from the beginning and should provide an impartial account of the incident. A nurse may be required to state whether or not an accident is a works injury. Sometimes this is obvious, and there is no problem. Occasionally, however, there may be times when it is not so easy to decide, e.g. a sudden hernia appearing after lifting, or back pain occurring after heavy or even light work.

Here the nurse should make the entry with the usual scrupulous care

and make a provisional note as to whether or not it is a works injury.
If the medical officer is available his advice could be sought. But having
decided as best she can, the decision whether to claim the higher rate of
benefit from the Social Security Office for those off sick with an injury
sustained at work is, of course, with the patient. If he is unable to work
as a result of a works injury, the patient completes parts A and B of the
National Health Service Medical Certificate and forwards this to the
Department of Health and Social Security. The claim is considered by
the Insurance Officer who asks the employer to confirm that the
accident did take place at work by means of a form B 176. Should the
patient decide to take action under common law at a later date, the
statement made at the time of injury will be vital to the patient, the
employer and the nurse concerned.

It must always be remembered that any entry may one day be used
in a court of law. Records have been known to be subjected to scrutiny
under a magnifying glass in the High Court.[6] The nurse needs to bear
this in mind whenever she makes an entry into a record book. It is a
serious duty to make a true and careful record. Memory can never be
relied upon. Any particular entry may mean a great deal to a patient,
the firm or the nurse.

Whenever action in law is taken there is an anxious time for all
concerned. The true facts, clearly recorded, will help everyone involved.
When a nurse is called upon to give evidence in a court of law, it helps
her self-confidence if her entry in the record also gives evidence of her
competence and professionalism.

To give examples as to the eventual use of records:

1. A contractor to a large firm had lime blown into his eyes on a
windy day in part of the works. He was treated by one of the nurses in
the firm. Expert care was given. After irrigation for some time the
patient was taken to the eye department of the local hospital where
further treatment was given.

A detailed record of his attendance was made. The nurse, however,
omitted to record the result of the Snellen's eye test which was carried
out before he left the department. When this man claimed against the
firm in common law, the entry in the record was needed, and vital
information as to his visual acuity was not available.

2. A contractor slipped on a patch of oil within part of the mills in
a large firm. He twisted his knee and reported to the occupational
health department. The nurse examined the knee, which was slightly
swollen, and applied a crepe bandage; she advised him to see his own
doctor if he had any trouble. The man decided he could manage to
return to work and he went back to his job and completed the shift.

The nurse made a careful and detailed record as to how the accident happened and the injury was sustained. When the contractor came to the occupational health department for information about his accident some 18 months later, he told the staff of the events which followed the incident. He finished his day's work, and by this time his knee was worse, and he visited his own doctor. After two operations and months of treatment he was now unable to kneel and so unable to do his own job. He was not a member of a Trade Union. The firm he had belonged to had been taken over by a larger concern and had moved its location. He was now unemployed, and bringing an action in common law against the firm where he was working when the accident occurred, claiming negligence because of the oil on the mill floor. The records kept on that occasion were very important.

3. A young apprentice had a severe epistaxis. This was treated by the nurse, who recorded only that 'the usual treatment' had been given, and that he returned to work. Three weeks later a shocked training officer told the occupational health department staff that this boy had died of leukaemia.

On questioning the nurse about this boy's attendance, she had indeed noticed the boy was very pale and had referred him to his own doctor, dealing expertly and kindly with the boy. But the record was not an adequate one, and did not tell the complete story.

Other papers in the Personal Health record will include:

notes made by a medical officer;
copies of medical certificates in date order;
letters from family doctor and hospital reports (these should be
    initialled by the nurse or medical officer before filling);
copies of any letters to family doctor and hospitals;
special screening examinations;
any refusal of treatment or advice forms signed by the patient.

(ii) Day Book (Daily Attendance Sheet)
Day Books have different titles in different health departments. The purpose of these books is to form a complete statistical record of all patients attending the occupational health department. The most satisfactory results from using these books are obtained when they are meticulously kept. The details of every patient attending can then be referred to at a later date. It should be possible to place sufficient confidence on their use that one could say with certainty that if the patient's name was not in the books, he had not been in the department as a patient.

Uses of the Day Book. The information may be needed perhaps years later for legal, medical or insurance purposes. It may be needed to protect or help the individual, the organisation, the nurse or doctor. By analysis, hazards to an employee or groups within the organisation may be highlighted and identified. Statistics may be compiled giving an overall picture of injury and disease, thus aiding prevention. It is a valuable indicator of the work of the department and could be used for research purposes into particular aspects of occupational health. Sometimes Day Books are used as described for the individual health record, but then information regarding attendances must be transferred from the book to the employee's personal health record and this duplicates work.

Compiling the Day Book. A type of ledger will be needed. The paper should be of a fairly good quality as it will be used and stored for long periods. It is essential that great care is taken in deciding what information will be needed and how the book should be designed before any large orders for books are placed, or printing done.

The entry for one patient necessitates so many details that the information could be spread over a double page. One well-tried method is to have a strong outer cover with loose leaf pages which can be detached after use. These pages are then transferred into similar binders with clear dates on the cover within the office area. Each binder would take six months' or a year's records. Confidentiality and ease of referral are aided by this method.

Storage of Day Books. In theory the records should be kept for at least three years, the time for a claim in common law to be made. In practice it has been found that referral to these records is needed for a variety of valid reasons long after this time. Confidentiality and security of these records are essential. If large quantities of records are involved, the feasibility of using microfilm methods of storage could be explored. This would facilitate storage, information, retrieval and confidentiality. Eventually disposal of the written record would be by shredding or burning.

The Information Needed. Whenever possible the entry in the Day Books should be begun when the patient enters the department.

Compiling Statistics. From the Day Book it is possible to retrieve information as to the number of patients attending for illness or injury.

By the use of a code it is possible to identify the types of injury sustained and the illnesses of patients reporting to the medical centre. The manual the *International Classification of Diseases*[7] provides an index of codes which can be used.

When this method is used, a code number is allocated to the entry in the Day Book, indicating the injury or disease of each patient. Great care needs to be taken in using the correct code for each individual attendance. If this is done less than thoroughly it may make the records of little statistical value.

Injury patterns can be built up. Figures can be obtained for the whole works, departments, groups, area, jobs or individuals, dependent on the information needed. Computer facilities will be needed for all but the smallest services. A programme will need to be devised to give the type of information required. Computer print-outs are, however, only as good as the information which is fed in. Scrupulous care is needed so that only correct information is used.

By having good records, knowing what type of information is needed, and devising the right programme, statistics may be obtained which warrant careful study and appraisal. Particular hazards may be pinpointed and preventive measures could be taken against industrial injury and disease. Research programmes may be warranted. Graphs or histograms may be used to make effective use of statistics. The information can often be more readily understood when simply displayed by these methods, rather than by tables of figures. This type of record is especially valuable when particular information is needed for a group of people, e.g. at a works council, to demonstrate reduction in eye injuries as a result of protective measures being implemented.

Treatment Card. This is a card which could be given to the patient in a very large establishment giving details of his illness or injury and the treatment given, signed by the nurse. The patient should bring this with him on each attendance. It is most useful for the patient to show this card to his foreman in the event of a works injury. It can be of help to him when filling in the accident report form. The card provides for continuity of care without prior referral to the individual record card which may accelerate the service being given. Should the patient go off sick whilst having treatment from the medical services he can show this card to his doctor. Although it is no substitute for the normal letter of referral by the nurse[8] (Whincup) it does give an indication of the treatment he has been having.

(iii) Group Records

It may well be very beneficial to keep a separate record of groups exposed to known hazards, even though the particular process involved may be one where the workers are not subject to statutory examination. Groups of workers at special risk could be those working with excessive noise, mineral oil, silica, asbestos, etc. The use of this record would be to ensure that employees at special risk were followed up. Enquiries could be made and individuals contacted if they did not attend for any screening measures. For example, some people working with mineral oil are protected by statutory medical examination.[9]

A list of names of employees who should attend for routine screening, e.g. drivers of any vehicles within the works, crane and fork-lift drivers, may be kept. A similar record could be kept for groups of patients at special risk because of their health, e.g. those with hypertension or obesity, who may need to be seen on a regular basis in the medical department.

A separate register may need to be kept for all employees immunised or vaccinated. This may be required, particularly in the National Health Service Occupational Health Departments where staff may have to work at short notice in areas where there are specific infections. This information may be urgently needed by those in charge of staffing arrangements. It may be of value too in an organisation where staff go abroad as part of their work, and need to have their immunisation programme kept up-to-date.

Sickness Absence Records. Medical certificates received in the department should be looked at and a note made in the Personal Health Record. Some certificates may give an indication of severe illness which may need to be followed up without delay.

Any visits to the patient whilst off sick at home or in hospital should be recorded in the Personal Health Record. The diagnoses may indicate an individual or group pattern of illness. Some medical certificates are, however, only useful to indicate that the person is off sick from work. They may be illegible or have a vague diagnosis, and thus have little further use.

Computer print-outs giving the length of any absence by employees are valuable. They identify people who are away for a significant length of time, and these may be followed up and further information sought as to the cause. They may also show up short spells of absence which may indicate personal or group problems. There may be other types of medical records kept in occupational health departments. It depends greatly on the needs of the organisation concerned. All medical records should be safeguarded with regard to confidentiality and security.

B. Environmental Records

Whatever the size or nature of the organisation, the occupational health nurse will be concerned with the working environment. It will greatly help her work and that of the occupational health team if environmental records are kept of all the various areas of the establishment. If the organisation is a large one, individual nurses may perhaps be delegated to be responsible for compiling environmental records for particular sections.

It is essential that records are kept up-to-date and that information can be extracted from them without delay. To make for ease of working, a check list could be devised, using for example the Royal College of Nursing Society of Occupational Health Nursing Leaflet no. 5 — Environmental Surveys. If a check list is compiled and set out in pro-forma sheets, these could be completed during the visits to the working area. This would be time-saving and would ensure that essential points were not omitted.

Essential points on the check list may include the following:

(a)   Date of the visit. Person contacted.

(b)   Name and telephone number of the area.

(c)   The site of the particular area; nearest access point (a plan or map is useful).

(d)   The hierarchy and names of individual managers, etc.

(e)   The product and process: type of work, skills needed.

(f)   Numbers and types of staff, shifts worked, disabled workers, trade unions.

(g)   Legislation applicable to the area.

(h)   Notice boards and telephones.

(i)   Standards of:
Cleanliness — housekeeping, state of decoration, walkways, disposal of waste.
Overcrowding.
Ventilation:[10] general, local, methods used, fume and dust extraction.
Heating:[10] type and methods used.
Floors: surfaces, drainage.
Lighting:[10] types, effectiveness.
Drinking water provisions.

Seating facilities.

Sanitary conveniences, washing facilities, clothing accommodation.

First Aid facilities: boxes, notices, emergency equipment.

Fire precautions: notices, alarms, extinguishers, fire doors, exits.

(j)   Specific Hazards such as:

Injury — possible causes, types of injury, machine guarding, methods of lifting, transport.

Chemical.[10]

Physical: thermal environment, noise, humidity, etc.

Biological.

Psychological.

Organisational: methods of payment, etc.

(k)   Protective clothing and safety equipment — available and in use.

A section could be left on the form for special comments by the nurse.

On return to the medical department the occupational health nurse should ensure that the relevant information has been noted, and the form completed. Any new hazard should be checked by means of Hazard Data Sheets or Guidance Notes from the Health and Safety Executive. Any new substances in use or cause for concern should be discussed with senior nursing or medical personnel. Discussion may be needed with the safety adviser or occupational hygienist. The completed check list of the visit should then be signed by the nurse and placed in the appropriate file; this should be clearly labelled and kept available for the occupational health team.

The specific areas of the organisation should be visited on a regular, routine basis. The record of the survey should help to ensure that the current hazards are known and controlled, and that individuals at risk are identified and monitored. The records of any monitoring procedures and type of instruments used should be clearly recorded.

These environmental records, up-to-date and available when needed, are most valuable and are a unique source of information to the occupational health nurse. They are particularly useful to nursing and medical staff who are new to the organisation.

C. Administrative Records

The smooth running of any medical department depends on soundly based organisation. Records can be used and systems devised to suit the particular needs of any department. These types of record could include:

1. Staff Records.
2. Departmental Records.
3. Correspondence.
4. Supplies and Ordering.
5. Drug Records.
6. Reports to Management.

1. Staff Records. These are required where a number of people work together. They should be treated as confidential information and kept under lock and key. The key should be held by the senior member of staff or her deputy.

Usually the staff records are begun with the original application form and a folder made which includes the professional information about the member of staff. It may be found useful to keep a record of such items as: date commenced duty, all overtime worked, number of days leave and dates, number of days off through illness, etc., courses attended, in-service training given, any certificates obtained. This might conveniently be kept in alphabetical order in an indexed book. This is useful information — often giving an indication as to progress. It may be used for assessments and in the event of references being required.

When a nurse leaves, the date and her reason for leaving, together with a short summary of her work, should be entered in the record. The records may be needed, perhaps many years after the writer has left, to give a reference for a nurse who may be quite unknown to the present holder of the post. Thus care and thought needs to be given to the compiling, writing and storage of these records. Memory of not very busy Sunday afternoons during training in the operating theatre served as a salutary lesson. The superintendent was known to keep a 'black book' with the names of nurses and their progress in the drawer of her desk. It was never locked. It was our dread and entertainment to read the latest entries, until one day we read 'Honesty doubtful' — without the name of the nurse!

It is often very useful to keep a record of all applicants for nursing posts. A waiting list can thus be formed and suitable candidates informed of an impending vacancy. A record could also be kept of staff willing and able to return in an emergency. In this way it is possible to develop a 'nurse bank' if agreement is obtained from management. Records of addresses and telephone numbers of staff should be kept up-to-date, and generally available in case of emergency.

2. Departmental Records. A loose-leaf book, or one with leaves of thin card instead of paper can be compiled to the advantage of the department, for items of information likely to be required regularly. A good index is needed, and the pages can be added to or removed as a topic changes. This is a good source of information and over the years an invaluable record can be collected.

It could include the addresses and telephone numbers of local voluntary organisations frequently used (e.g. Marriage Guidance Council); or details of how to reach the local hospitals and dental school for those who do not know the area; how to obtain various supplies — which supplier may be called on for vaccines, etc., when other sources have none available. This is a quick and easy form of reference which can be used by all staff when necessary.

Another method may be to put the information on cards — the size of a large post-card — and store in alphabetical order in a plastic flip-top box. The advantage of this method is that a card can be removed and another inserted very easily.

Records of addresses and telephone numbers needed in an emergency can best be located by the telephones used. Continual up-dating to ensure accuracy is needed. The medical department should keep records of all accidents occurring to members of staff or patients whilst in the medical department.

Usually the same type of record is kept as is used in the rest of the organisation. Two copies may be made, the top copy sent to the Safety Department or Personnel Department. The carbon copy is retained for reference within the department. The accidents can then be investigated and prevention assisted.

All complaints, unless of a minor nature and dealt with straight away to the satisfaction of everyone concerned, should be recorded. A record of the incident, the action taken and how the incident was resolved should be made. The use of this record ensures that all complaints are brought to the attention of senior staff and they are effectively dealt with. This record should be part of a definite complaints procedure, in accordance with good working practice.

Information for nurses should also be available within the medical department for the nurse to refer to if in any doubt about her duties. These could take the form of Standing Orders, which should be drawn up by the senior nurse and Medical Officer, with agreement by the staff. They should be read and understood by all staff including new nurses. The Standing Orders should be revised regularly, and signed by the nurses. Management should be in agreement with this record.

There could also be available a Procedure Manual — any set methods of doing a particular nursing task. This also should be up-to-date.

Additionally, a Disaster Plan should be available for a serious emergency and the staff should be familiar with this record.

A record could be kept of the time any emergency call for First Aid assistance was received, and the time of arrival at the incident, and arrival at hospital. This record of timing helps to pinpoint any delays. It can be used in the event of any complaint of delay.

Where there is shift working within the department, or any break in the continuity of staffing, a Report Book may be found valuable. Where such a book is kept, the reasons for entries should be well thought out. Report books have been encountered which served no useful purpose! Information from the Day Book had been duplicated resulting in wastage of the nurse's time.

Entries could be made to draw attention to the Medical Officer, senior sister or shift staff of exceptional circumstances, such as where serious or fatal accidents or illness have occurred, and whether or not the relatives had been contacted; notification of a new hazard within the organisation; progress report on any patients recently taken to hospital with severe illness or injury; where a standing order authorising the use of drugs in an emergency has been implemented, and such medication given to a patient by the nurse on duty; any fault in equipment, so that this could be rectified; details of any patients refusing to accept advice or treatment, together with a record signed by the patient to this effect, e.g. deciding to drive his own car home when not well.

All entries should be dated and signed. The report should be initialled after reading. In short, it is a means of conveying information which is out of the normal run of events. It could help with communication and the smooth running of the department.

It is useful to keep an Inventory Record, a simple record of equipment and furniture within the department. The list can be compiled room by room.

It is useful to do a check yearly to ensure that items are present in the department, and that they are in good order. Where necessary, items may be repaired, replaced or discarded. It is a good plan to replace items which may well have depreciated in value. Electrical equipment in particular should be checked with regard to replacement. When changes are made in an inventory the records should be amended accordingly. Surplus equipment can be disposed of by arrangement with the supplies officer. This item can then be deleted from the inventory.

Minor items of equipment, e.g. plastic or polypropathene goods may be so cheap that it is not worth the cost of time involved to check on these items. The inventories should be kept in folders, and signed after a check has been done.

Where equipment is subject to regular servicing, all details need to be kept in a book especially for this purpose. When the item has been serviced and is in use again, this date should also be entered. The use of these records ensures that all equipment subject to a regular check is in good working order, and is not overdue for attention.

In a large medical department it is often a good plan to keep a note of when walls were painted or washed. This ensures that none are left, and that work can be done in rotation.

3. Records of Correspondence. An orderly filing system is essential. Dale Carnegie once wrote about a millionaire, who attributed his success in business to the fact that he never put anything down, he put it away!

A copy of each letter sent from the department should be kept. Items needing to be kept together should be pinned or stapled; paper clips often slip or take in another piece of paper. Out-of-date correspondence should be cleared from the files when no longer needed.

4. Supplies Record. A business-like system should be implemented for ease of work with regard to obtaining supplies. Order books with a carbon copy retained give information with regard to items ordered, together with dates and order number. Where these are medical purchases or items with unusual terms these entries are best ordered by block capitals — so they are clearly read by the typist putting out the order. This minimises any errors in delivery.

Where an item is one which is recurring or is regularly used, a card system may perhaps be implemented with the supplies officer. This is sometimes known as a 'travelling requisition'. When items need to be ordered the relevant cards can be selected from a small desk file, the amount of the items required entered and the cards sent to the supplies officer. The advantages of this system are that:

(i)   it is simple to operate;

(ii)   duplication of information is avoided, as all relevant information, including stores bin number, is already on the card;

(iii)   the amount of any particular item, e.g. First Aid dressings, drugs used, etc., can be seen at a glance. Stock control is aided;

(iv)   when the items are received the cards can be signed and put away until they are needed again.

Delivery notes, statements of account, and receipts should always be dealt with promptly. This aids the business side of the organisation and helps with budgetary control. Any relevant receipts should be filed and stored in dated files. The advice of the supplies officer should be sought as to the eventual date of disposal of these records.

5. Drug Records. A record should be kept of all drugs ordered and received. Drugs dispensed to patients should be noted in the Day Book and on the Personal Health Record.

Under the Medicines Act 1968 there are three classes of medicines: General Sales List Medicines (GSL); Pharmacy Medicines (P); and Prescription only Medicines (POM). There is no legal requirement to keep records of GSL or Pharmacy Medicines, but it is good practice to keep a record of the usage of these items. Prescription only Medicine records must, however, be kept for two years.

The Medicines Act 1968 Part III Regulations permit a Registered or Enrolled Nurse to order in writing, supply or administer Pharmacy Medicines and Prescription only Medicines providing there is a written general instruction by a doctor as to the circumstances in which the POM of the description in question are to be used in the course of the Occupational Health Scheme.

There should be a record of the written general instruction by the medical officer, duly signed by the nursing staff in agreement with this instruction. This record should be up-dated regularly in accordance with good occupational health nursing practice, as recommended by the Royal College of Nursing.

Controlled Drugs (under the Misuse of Drugs Act 1971 (The Misuse of Drugs Regulations 1973 SI 797) fall into four categories: (Schedule 4 has no therapeutic use).

(i) Controlled Drugs marked 'CD Inv' (Schedule 1):[11] these drugs include Codeine Linctus B.P. or Kaolin and Morphine mixture B.P.C. These contain controlled drugs in such small amounts that they will not produce dependence or harm if misused. No register is needed but the drug invoice must be kept for two years.

Medicines under Schedule 1 may be either Prescription Only Medicines but not fully Controlled Drugs (CD Inv POM) or Pharmacy Medicines and not fully controlled Drugs CD Inv P).

(ii) Controlled Drugs marked 'CD' (Schedule 2): these include the opiates such as morphine. Any Schedule 2 drugs must be checked and recorded on receipt by the sister-in-charge or her deputy. These records should be checked regularly to ensure they balance. All Schedule 2 drugs should be checked by another nurse and both signatures recorded.

If any drugs are to be destroyed this can only be done in the presence of a person authorised by the Secretary of State and the quantity of drugs destroyed must be entered in the Register of Controlled Drugs and signed by the authorised person. A special Register is kept; the form of the Register is the same as that of the repealed Dangerous Drugs Act. The Register is kept for two years from the date of the last entry. Medicines under Schedule 2 are all Prescription only Medicines and Fully Controlled Drugs (CD POM).

(iii) Controlled Drugs marked 'CD No Register' (Schedule 3): these include a small number of minor stimulant drugs or other drugs which are not thought to be so harmful as Schedule II. A Register is not required.

Under the Dangerous Drugs Regulations, 1953, there is a group authority by the Secretary of State to State Registered Nurses and Certified First Aid men at certain mines, quarries and factories to be in possession of and to administer morphine. Although this legislation has been repealed this group authority is still statutory, but this is being revised and brought under the Misuse of Drugs Act 1971. This authority is given by the authorised Medical Officer, who is a registered medical practitioner employed for medical supervision of employees at the factory. Where this group authority is in operation, a record of this written authority must be kept and should be signed by the State Registered Nurses and Certificated First Aid men duly authorised.

6. Reports to Management. These will depend on the type of organisation. Management may request the occupational health nurse for a report on a particular topic and perhaps on a regular basis. This could well happen with regard to any area which has caused concern, e.g. works kitchens.

A dated, impersonal record of any survey could be given, with suggestions for improvements. It is essential that all the people concerned should have a copy of the report for reference. An annual report should be made to management, with a record of the work and activity of the medical department over the past year. The record should be available to the medical department staff as it will be of value in assessing the work of the department.

Conclusion

These then are some of the records which may be found in a medical department. Properly kept they are a most useful tool of the occupational health nurse. There are perhaps two golden rules to remember out of all the information given. Records should be clear and they should be correct.

Notes

1. Central Health Services Council, *The Standardisation of Hospital Medical Records* (HMSO, London, 1965).
2. A. Elliot *et al.*, 'Complete Conversion of Health Centre Records to A4 Size', *British Medical Journal*, vol.12 (1975), p.773.
3. R.J. Holdich, 'The Importance of Patient Care Records', *Nursing Times* (13 July 1978), p.1159.
4. M. Gentle, 'A Transfer Form for Use Between Hospitals and Industrial Medical Departments', *Injury*, vol.3, no.4 (April 1972).
5. J.C.G. Pearson and D. Radwanski, 'Principles of Design of Occupational Health Records', *Journal of the Society of Occupational Medicine*, vol.24 (1974), pp.17-24.
6. A.L. Gwynne, 'The Legal Importance of Nursing Notes', *Nursing Times* (13 July 1978), p.1162.
7. World Health Organisation (Geneva), *International Classification of Diseases Manual of the International Statistical Classification of Diseases, Injuries and Causes of Death*, vol. II, alphabetical, (published in Great Britain by HMSO).
8. M. Whincup, 'Legal Aspects of Occupational Health Nursing', *Nursing Times* (9 August 1973), p.127.
9. Certain workers with mineral oil have a statutory medical examination; those working under the Patent Fuel Manufacture Regulations 1972 and the Mule Spinning (Health) Regulations 1972.
10. Note that the records of any monitoring procedures and type of instrument used should be clearly recorded.
11. C.E. Hay, *Medicines and Poisons Guide* (Pharmaceutical Press, 1978), pp.19-23.

Further Reading

Rcn Society of Occupational Health Nursing Information Leaflets: no.10 'Disclosure of Information under Statutory Provisions – Confidentiality and the Occupational Health Nurse'; no.11 'Duties and Responsibilities of Occupational Health Nurses : Notes of guidance and the duties and responsibilities of Occupational Health Nurses under the provisions of the Medicines Act 1968 and subsequent regulations'.
D. Ross, 'A Medical Record System', *Occupational Health*, vol.27, no.12 (December 1975), pp.516-23.
P.J. Taylor and A.W. Gardner, 'Treatment Services' in R.S.F. Schilling (ed.), *Occupational Health Practice* (Butterworths, London, 1973), pp.159-68.

5 HEALTH SUPERVISION

Peter Holgate

It is stated[1] that health supervision is one of the nurse's functions in occupational health. This, at times, has to be seen as an overt exercise as there are many people at work who are not the slightest bit interested in their own health and others who would regard the nurse's help as an intrusion into their privacy. This does not mean that health supervision in an organisation should be abandoned; on the contrary, persistent efforts may be rewarded especially if a previously unknown health problem is identified.

For the purpose of this chapter, consider that health supervision is an ongoing process in the form of health examinations, biological measurements and any other arrangements necessary to maintain the health of the worker. The word supervision cannot be used narrowly, because often the nurse is not involved in the overall strategy of some particular health care project e.g. workers handling asbestos, but may be one of a team, each completing a particular facet of the project.

Management Policy

Before looking at the different work groups to consider *who* needs health supervision, one must look at the management policy of the organisation.

What is the policy? Is it written down? Who wrote it? The first stage for the nurse is to find out and this is not always an easy exercise. In some companies this may only be found in her job description, i.e. 'Will carry out pre-employment examinations for new staff'. At least it will be discovered that there is a pre-employment examination policy and, in some large organisations, that may be the sole job for which the nurse is employed. Other organisations may have evolved their policy as to the result of the particular skills and interests of previous medical and nursing staff and a nurse may have inherited a range of examinations that are not relevant to today's needs but may be difficult to discontinue, e.g. some workers still demand the medical examination that was required under the Chromium Plating Regulations 1931, but no longer required under the Chromium Plating Regulations 1973, when environmental monitoring of the chromic acid tank is undertaken.

Now under the Health and Safety at Work etc., Act 1974 Section 2(3) management has a duty to write a health and safety policy. In the early policy writings, some companies either failed to mention health, or made some glib overall comment that in reality meant nothing. From 1978 the Chief Inspector of Factories directed his Inspectors' attention[2] to these policy statements and required companies to rewrite them if necessary, spelling out precise details as required by Section 2(3) of the Act. If the policy has got to be rewritten then it is to be hoped that the Occupational Health Unit will be consulted and for those nurses working alone, it is professionally irresponsible to allow somebody else to write a policy that has implications for the daily work load, without being involved in the consultations.

Also to be considered either initially, when deciding the policy, or subsequently, if a potential hazard is identified, is consultation with shop floor representatives. It can often invite rebuff to try to institute a procedure, however well intentioned it is, without having involved the work force.

It is possible to detect certain progressive diseases at a pre-symptomatic stage by the use of common biological tests. This could be useful in accident prevention, e.g. by periodic testing of all drivers within an organisation whether they drive lorries, cranes, fork-lift trucks or even mechanical work savers. However, there is a natural fear of what will happen to a worker if an abnormality is detected: will he lose his job, will he lose bonuses, etc ? To prevent this anxiety there should be discussions with workers' representatives, and a clear policy established.

Procedure Manual

Once a policy has been laid down by management then procedures need to be written down and put together as a procedure manual. The act of writing down the procedure, especially the different stages of documentation, will often be helpful in identifying any flaws in the procedure — for example, who else, in addition to Personnel, should be notified when an individual is accepted as a new employee?

Many nurses query the value of doing this but it should be remembered that they are not always present; they may have been taken ill or have gone on holiday. Whatever the reason for absence, it is professionally responsible to leave the department in some semblance of order so that whoever replaces the nurse temporarily will know the procedure required for the employee who needs an examination for a driving permit, for instance, or before becoming a welder, or whatever is special to the organisation.

Health Examinations

One aspect of health supervision is conducting health examinations. A point of clarification should be the distinction between health and medical examinations. Medical examinations are carried out by doctors but health examinations may be carried out by nurses or health technicians.

There is no legal reason why nurses cannot carry out health examinations, provided the individual employee agrees to submit to the procedure. During the nurse's general training she is taught a variety of biological tests for measurements, e.g. urine testing, measurement of weight, etc. She is also taught the parameters of normality and, therefore, if an abnormality is present she should be able to recognise it.

Before carrying out health examinations there should be an agreed procedure of what to do when an abnormality occurs. The nurse should work on a pass rather than a fail basis. It is professionally undesirable for a nurse to make the decision that a prospective employee is declined on medical grounds. This must be a management decision as the health service can only advise management. Even when a report is received from a medical adviser (be it the individual's general practitioner or company doctor) the advice must be worded so that the diagnosis is not disclosed, but management is clearly aware that there is a health problem, i.e. an individual with chronic bronchitis would have the recommendation to management 'not to work in a dusty atmosphere'. If management do not have a suitable job because all their work is dusty, then they will decline the applicant. The situation also occurs, when management wants a particular individual because of his skill and expertise, and in spite of an undesirable health risk will ignore all objections in order to secure those skills.

Health examinations can be subdivided into *pre-placement* or *periodic*.

Pre-placement Health Examinations

A lot of people still use the expression 'pre-employment'; unfortunately this has the connotation of a 'hire and fire' situation. The facts may be that this is so, but in occupational health one should be thinking positively in terms of placing individuals in work compatible with their physical and psychological needs.

To undertake this type of examination it is necessary to know the physical and psychological demands of all jobs within an organisation. This knowledge can only be obtained by nurses who have access to all work areas in the organisation, and have studied people at work. In large organisations where there could be many demands on the Health Unit, it may be necessary to assess priorities among the working groups. What type of pre-placement examination is required for which particular job? The ideal may be to establish base lines for every worker, but the practicalities are often different. Is it worth carrying out expensive, time-consuming examinations on large numbers of people when they might not even start work? Or should all those who start, and have left the job by the end of the first week be examined? These may be a few of the criteria that have to be considered when establishing a policy within an organisation.

This has led to the policy in some companies of grading certain jobs with particular health criteria.

(a) Health Questionnaire. All workers on application for work fill in a health questionnaire, which should be returned to the Health Unit, not the Personnel Department, in a sealed envelope marked 'Confidential'. Anybody disclosing an obvious health problem can be requested to visit the Health Unit. There is a great deal of mistrust of this method as the papers might be read by anybody unless a good procedure is established.

(b) Health Interview. Certain categories of work may require a more detailed examination or an individual health questionnaire may warrant investigation. This examination may be carried out by a nurse and usually consists of a recognised range of screening tests including measurement of height, weight, visual acuity, pulse, blood pressure and urine testing. Sometimes a known hazard requires a special test, e.g. audiometry, vitalograph or cardiograph.

(c) Medical Examination. Certain occupations may require by statutory law (see Chapter 4), or company policy, that the examination should be carried out by a doctor. Also included in this category should be those individuals where health problems have been revealed to the nurses, and she has referred to the doctor for further consultation.

An area of anxiety is the lack of a reliable form of psychological testing. This was highlighted when the Department of Health and Social Security issued a reminder that doctors should have pre-employment medical examinations on appointment.[3] This followed publicity after a homicide in a children's ward. There are a wide variety of psychological tests that are used in industry in selection for a variety of occupations. Among these some will identify possible neurosis but not many will help identify those with psychotic disease.

Periodic Health Examinations

These examinations, although they may often only be interviews, occur in a variety of forms, usually dependent on the organisational policy.

1. Return to Work After Sickness/Injury Absence

This is an extremely helpful form of health supervision which requires a personal knowledge of the industry coupled with good clinical knowledge. Various organisations have different policies. The important point is that a system is established of seeing *everybody* who has been absent for a defined period, whether it is one day or three days, or longer. It always appears easier to establish a return to work health policy for weekly paid workers, but salaried workers are more difficult to involve within a system; their illnesses are never the same as mortal man's!

With the increasing distances that people commute to work, it is impossible to expect an employee's family doctor to have knowledge of work conditions or company policies for alternative work. Again, for a variety of reasons, some employees try to persuade their doctors to allow a return to work before they are fully fit (although if one believed everything in the national press the impression might be gained that the reverse is true and that workers persuade their doctor to keep them off work longer than is necessary).

If the nurse is running a department where workers do not report back after periods of sickness absence, then it will be difficult to claim health supervision as a function of the occupational health unit.

To be able to fulfil the aims of occupational health some knowledge is required of the frequency and cause of illness amongst individuals and groups of workers. When seeing workers on return to work, one occasionally picks up an individual who has suddenly started having frequent spells of absence, after a long record of good health. Sometimes the condition may be as described on the medical certificate, but often there may be other problems especially within a working group, reflecting stress, anxiety or bad inter-personal relationships. These are aspects, occasionally non-medical, that have a strong influence on the mental health of employees.

If there is a doctor, either full or part-time, then the nurse should establish with him a 'return to work' policy before consulting with management and workers' representatives. There are various factors to be considered.

   (a) Company policy on length of uncertified sickness absence, i.e. are workers allowed to be off three days or less without submitting a medical certificate?

   (b) Should all works injuries be seen irrespective of length of absence?

   (c) What period of absence elapses before cases are seen by the works doctor, three weeks, four weeks, three months?

   (d) Are there any clinical conditions that should always be seen, irrespective of the period of absence (for example, food handlers suffering from diarrhoea)?

2. Rehabilitation After Injury or Illness

Another aspect of health supervision is ensuring that any individual who has an injury or illness is suitably rehabilitated. This does not necessarily mean that an individual has to lose time before he can be rehabilitated. Apparently simple injuries are sometimes the most painful and prevent resumption of normal working, e.g. bruising of a thumbnail with subungual haematoma can prevent the firm gripping of hand tools. Alternatively, consideration has to be given after treatment. If a wound dressing has been applied to a finger of a kitchen worker then it would be inappropriate for the worker to return to the usual job and get the dressing soaking wet; or if a local anaesthetic has been instilled in a patient's eye then it must be covered with a pad before returning to work, and the nurse must ensure that the job to which he returns is safe for the employee.

   Any individual who has been placed in modified work as a result of accident or illness must have a time limit placed on the recommendation and, at the end of the limit, the individual should be seen again to assess progress. Obviously the review period will vary with the condition, depending on whether it is acute or chronic. The review can be as short as daily, extending to seeing an individual once a year.

   Among the problems of having a rehabilitation policy, will be that of the individual presenting a medical certificate 'Fit for light work'. The same certificate can have different meanings to the worker, his supervisior, his workmates and to the staff of an occupational health unit. The nurse will need to establish the company policy in this matter; local agreements especially involving bonus and piece work payments might exclude any worker who cannot achieve 100 per cent work performance. Again, there may be only a limited number of jobs designated for light work and these may be filled by other workers. The management may feel that a medical certificate stating 'Fit for light work' means a change of job, a view that may be shared by the worker himself. The situation requires an accurate appraisal of the demands of the job and an assessment of the employee's ability. In many cases it can be shown that the existing work is within the individual's capability. Management also have the impression that people on light work are not performing efficiently whereas intelligent placing of a worker can often mean that nearly 100 per cent output can be achieved, as witnessed by the work performance of some severely disabled workers.

Lastly, there are the attitudes of the worker's colleagues themselves to consider. These attitudes can span the whole range of the spectrum from anxiety about having to 'carry' an individual who cannot make his full contribution to the team, to concern and excessive shielding of a worker by his mates when sometimes it would have been better for the individual to stand alone.

3. Request by an Individual for an Examination

This is probably the easiest situation to classify under health supervision, but can be extremely important and demanding of clinical and inter-personal skills.

The worker may present at the Health Unit requesting an examination when fears have been aroused either from an item in the press or on television about e.g. asbestos, concern about hair dyes, or from conversation with workmates about particular work processes that they are currently using or may have used in their previous work experience. The clinical aspects should be considered as sometimes an employee may have already consulted his own doctor.

Professional guidelines need to be established with the Occupational Medical Adviser as to when, and in what circumstances, an examination can be offered to employees and what should be the contact between patient, his general practitioner and the staff of the occupational health unit.

4. Request by Management

There are many situations when management may request the staff of the Health Unit to examine a worker. It may be a formal situation arising from various conditions of employment, such as prior to promotion or transfer from hourly paid to salary status, or as a condition for entering the company's pension fund.

The informal situation occurs when supervision send a worker to the Health Unit either because the worker says he is unable to do a certain job due to a health problem, or because supervision are unhappy about an employee's work performance. These can cause some of the trickiest inter-personal problems.

First, there is the worker who feels that he cannot do the job to which he has been assigned. There may be an obvious health problem and one may confidently advise management to this effect. Occasions will occur when the nurse cannot find an obvious health problem, but in the interim may advise management that a change of job is desirable until the employee has been examined by the company's doctor, or his general practitioner. However, the nurse will lose integrity with the organisation if it becomes known that it is easy to get taken off unpleasant work by visiting the occupational health department. Situations will arise where it is necessary to take a stand and advise management *and* the worker that it is the opinion of the occupational health staff that the worker is fit for his usual work.

Secondly, management may be unhappy about an individual sickness absence record, or lack of achievement of full work performance. The situation may be made difficult when a worker presents himself to the Health Unit, unaware of the reason for his attendance as he has been sent by his supervisor, usually after a telephone call to the Health Unit. The nurse must ensure that the worker knows why he is present and, if any examination is being considered, then he should be invited to submit to the examination, otherwise the staff may be technically committing an assault. Society has not yet reached the position when individuals can be forced to have an examination, in spite of what is apparently felt by some managements.

Information to management should be carefully couched in words that do not give any indication of a clinical condition. This can be very difficult, especially with problems such as alcoholism. The Health Unit should make every effort not to be associated with company disciplinary problems.

5. Workers with Known Progressive Disease
Within any working group there will be individuals who are suffering from one of the diseases that often have periods of remission, but will eventually create disabilities that may make working difficult, for example, cardiac or rheumatic problems, osteo-arthritis or diabetes. They do not warrant frequent attendances at the Health Unit but, depending on the degree of disability, they should be seen at least

annually. If deterioration is occurring then they can be seen more frequently and long term plans considered for work placement. It is sometimes easier to care for these people by visiting them at their place of work, when the nurse is ostensibly carrying out some other function.

Immunisation

As was stated at the beginning of this chapter, health supervision is not just about health examinations. Where workers may be exposed to infection because of their work, or may have to travel to countries where certain diseases are endemic, then immunisation will be one method of maintaining their health status. In particular, immunisation may be offered to workers who travel abroad for their holiday, but it is essential that the company product is protected, as in the food industry.

The biggest group of workers who use protection are those whose work is involved continuously with microbiological hazards and this explains why immunisation programmes provide a major part of the work load of hospital Occupational Health Services. Because of the continuous exposure to this form of hazard, and because of the mobility of this work force from one employee to another, it would seem reasonable for nurses, doctors and medical laboratory staff to have a personal record card of their immunisation status.

Another major infection is tetanus. The Health Unit of any occupation, where there is risk of a puncture wound from soil contaminated objects, such as with agricultural workers, gardeners, firemen and refuse collectors, may have as part of their health policy a programme to keep tetanus immunisation up to date.

Special Groups

It has been shown that health supervision is a combination of health examination, immunisation, epidemiology and possibly health education, particularly when the Health Unit gives instruction about a known health hazard. The different working groups within an organisation, to whom health supervision may be provided, are best classified according to statutory and non-statutory.

Statutory

The examination is carried out either by an Employment Medical Adviser or an 'appointed doctor'. The most frequent examinations are for those regulations affecting lead, ionising radiations, compressed air and chemicals. Many of these processes have been revolutionised by technology. The regulations still exist, but either the hazard is well controlled or the form of examination is not reliable; for example, the law only requires a three-monthly haemoglobin estimation for lead workers, whereas most Health Units involved in this examination also measure the serum lead and other blood levels.

Non-Statutory

There are other work processes that have known health hazards but there are no regulations requiring any form of health examination. Good employers and Health Units have introduced their own forms of biological and environmental monitoring, either following Codes of Practice published by the Government, or devised within their own industry.

1. Special Hazards

Examples of the different health hazards may be shown by the method of monitoring.

(a) Biological Monitoring

(i) Urine sampling for workers working with trichloroethylene and benzene.

(ii) Blood sampling for workers not covered by regulations, but still using lead compounds particularly in the car industry and workers using organo-phosphorus compounds for agricultural use.

(iii) Measurement of respiratory function for employees working with Bacillus Subtilis in the manufacture of biological detergents, for those working with asbestos and welders who are at risk from inhalation of nitrous fumes.

(b) Environmental Monitoring

This may be in the form of noise measurement, the measurement of chromic acid mist in electroplating works, or the use of gas detector tubes for carbon monoxide, hydrogen sulphide or methane levels.

2. Catering Workers

Although the Food Hygiene Regulations 1970 require an employee to notify an employer if he is suffering from a group of gastro-intestinal infections or staphylococcal infection there is no obligation for the employer to have any statement of health status when commencing work.

In the food manufacturing industry, those companies concerned with the public image of their product usually have some form of health supervision of the workers. Far-sighted management in industries not involved with food manufacture, have realised that the works canteen, although only employing a small proportion of the labour force, has the ability to cripple the company if there is a major outbreak of food poisoning. Food poisoning is a far from remote possibility as evidenced by the yearly increasing incidence.

Ideally, health supervision will require some form of examination before the individual commences employment and there will need to be follow up in the work situation.Co-operation with the catering supervisor in this matter is essential and a policy should be agreed on as to whether all catering workers are seen after sickness absence and, for example, whether there should be stool culture for new employees and those returning to work after a gastro-intestinal upset, especially if it occurred whilst abroad.

3. Drivers

There are very few organisations that do not have employees involved in some form of driving either externally as chauffeurs, lorry drivers or sales representatives, or internally, as crane or fork-lift truck drivers.

For those organisations whose drivers operate heavy goods vehicles, English law only requires a medical declaration when the licence is being granted and no further medical examination until the driver is aged 60 years. The onus is on the driver to declare any change in his health status should it occur earlier.

There is a tendency for organisations to introduce some form of health examination as company policy for its drivers. This is designed not only as health supervision of the individual driver, but of the rest of the work force. There cannot be anything more hazardous than a fork-lift driver with defective vision, careering around a congested shop with a bulky load.

The policy needs to include guidelines on the frequency of the examination. There seems little point in yearly examination of everybody otherwise the examination can fall into similar disrepute like the examination of young adults before the Employment Medical Advisory Service Act 1972. The average period appears to be every 3-5 years up to the age of 45 years, reducing in frequency up to about 55 years old, and then annually thereafter.

A useful document that gives valuable guidelines on the relationship between driving and various clinical conditions is 'Medical Aspects of Fitness to Drive', published by the Medical Commission on Accident

Prevention.

Increasing public concern about the transport by road of oil, gas and hazardous chemicals, may lead to the Health and Safety Commission laying down standards on the frequency of such examinations. What will be needed for companies involved in transport is a policy that will cover the situation when a worker can no longer drive because of health reasons.

4. Executives

It may be the company policy for senior staff to have an annual medical examination. In this age of fringe benefits, health care has been welcomed by management although doubt has been cast on the value of this form of examination. Nonetheless, it is an opportunity once a year for very busy people to consider their own health. What has to be remembered is that an adverse decision made by a manager with a health problem can have far reaching effects on the company and its employees.

So far, this chapter has tried to identify the extent to which an occupational health nurse can apply herself to health supervision within the work place. It may be argued that this is her true role and it can be extremely satisfying to function effectively.

Before rushing into taking on all aspects of health supervision, some thought must be given to other factors. A great range of health supervision practices may be the ideal, but in a real world less than the ideal is possible. There is a physical limit to the amount of work that an individual can perform and one must, of necessity, establish priorities. Is it more important to give every employee a pre-employment health examination or is the nurse's time better spent identifying health risks within particular working groups by regular visits to the workplace? Can it be shown that health examination of individuals reduces the accident rate, sickness absence level or labour turnover? What is the true cost of pre-placement health examinations when the time involved, overheads of the department for the time spent carrying out the examination, cost of equipment, secretarial costs and the cost of sending for applicants is included, especially when many potential employees never start after examination, or have left by the end of the first week? Would it be better to have the health screening during the probationary month? Can the role in health supervision influence the course of any disease that may be detected by routine health screening? There are some authorities who would claim that pre-symptomatic testing does not alter the outcome of the disease whether it is for cancer of the breast or hypertension.

What is necessary is that the nurse has a rationale for action, that the matter has been well thought out and that a policy has been evolved.

Notes

1. *Guide to Occupational Health Nursing Service* (Rcn, London, 1975).

2. Health and Safety Executive, Manufacturing and Service Industries, Annual Report of H.M. Factory Inspectorate (HMSO, London, 1976).

3. Restricted memorandum, Department of Health and Social Security DS/84/73 and Chief Medical Officer, letter dated 27 November, 1973.

6 HEALTH EDUCATION

Jean Allsopp

Unlike other environments where the nurse's role is specifically one of restoring health, in industry the occupational health nurse primarily carries out a role of prevention of ill health, by endeavouring to ensure the well-being of the employee and a safe working environment.

To do this the nurse must constantly be educating and showing the need for such education, in practically everything that she does. She may have to possess much determination in order to achieve the desired results; in some circumstances only tactful but firm persistence may convince worker, management or union that ingrained habits or procedures should be changed. In large companies where an organised Training Department exists, the role of the nurse in teaching is made considerably easier as she is expected to participate and will receive in return the necessary co-operation. Where no Training Manager is employed the nurse must use her initiative, perhaps by approaching the Personnel Department with a view to establishing group teaching sessions, while promoting health on an individual basis from the Occupational Health Department.

This chapter will deal with the health education needs throughout industry, showing the needs of people at different ages, or from different cultures. Methods of teaching will be discussed and use of equipment will be included. Finally the nurse's own training to prepare her for her role as a teacher will be explored, and sources of assistance in the planning of her programme will be given.

What is Health Education?

In an industrial situation health education could be considered as the educating of the employee, employer and unions in all aspects of health, to enable each to protect his own or his colleagues' optimum physical and mental well-being and to ensure a safe working situation. However, it is unlikely that the occupational health nurse will be confined to the industrial situation only, in her efforts to promote health — the employees for whom she provides the service will expect her to advise them also on home or community health problems when requested. Nurses experienced in this field know that many an employee is given inadequate basic instructions from hospitals or doctors when coping with illness in the family and they will often turn to the company nurse for guidance. So the nurse's role is one of health promotion in its widest aspect, domestic, occupational and communal.

Health education begins in childhood with Health Visitors who call at individual homes to see parents and who teach in schools. It is carried out in hospital clinics and wards all the time by general or specialist nurses. After retirement it may be continued by Geriatric Health Visitors. However, between school leaving age and retirement there is little provision made for such education in normal daily life; this period accounts for approximately one third of the average person's life. Occupational health nurses are therefore in the unique position of having a fairly settled audience for considerable lengths of time, enabling the nurse to establish a long term programme.

In considering her programme the nurse must first decide *whom* she is going to educate, *what* health topics she should promote, *when* she will do it and *how* it will be done.

Who Benefits From Health Education?

There will be no individual, or group of employees, that will neither need nor benefit from health education, and they could be considered in some of the following groups.

New staff need to be orientated into the company routine and health requirements. The nurse has a golden opportunity in this instance to establish health instruction and to explain her role within the company, by assisting at the weekly Induction Training that most companies hold for new staff during the first week of appointment.

Young people need educating into a responsible approach to life, in a non-critical manner. At school leaving age they are careless of safety and health and frequently experiment with drugs, alcohol and sex as they approach adulthood. They will often turn to a known company nurse for advice on subjects that they would fear to discuss with parents, subjects such as suspected venereal disease, contraception or how to remedy such conditions as acne as they become more conscious of their appearance.

Women also have special problems, possibly the most common being diet. It is very important in pregnancy to maintain an adequate protein and calcium intake, to avoid excess carbohydrate (and therefore a fat baby) and to control constipation and habits such as smoking. Women with husbands and families will often neglect their own nutrition when finances are limited in order to provide for the family adequately. The need for cervical cytology and breast self examination is very important after childbearing and from the menopause onwards. The problems associated with menopausal hormone imbalance also need to be explained in order to help women to cope with this major change in their lives.

Immigrant workers have very special problems which require education, problems such as a different approach to personal hygiene and the use of the European type of pedestal toilet — as opposed to the Asian type which is sunk into the ground. Some immigrant women also practise primitive and unhygienic forms of contraception leading to salpingitis and occlusion of the uterine tubes, so advice on this subject is needed. Nutrition may present difficulties due to religious restrictions, or where a company accepts refugees the case may be one of malnutrition. Clothing is important where loose robes may become tangled in machinery or the wearing of turbans interferes with the use of safety equipment such as helmets and goggles. It may be necessary to encourage adequate clothing to be worn in winter. The nurse can help foreign workers to absorb the new culture by careful and tactful orientation.

Shift workers may need educating into regular sleeping or eating habits, especially where a married couple work opposite shifts in order to care for children. This generally means that the wife works during the day, and the husband cares for the children when he should be sleeping in preparation for his night job. Such a situation causes much domestic stress, in addition to affecting job performance due to lack of rest.

Executives, as members of senior management, are subject to much strain with projected forecasts that must be met, the entertaining of clients, or sales promotions which often involve international travel. The nurse might teach methods of relaxation, control of alcohol and smoking and encourage regular eating habits. Explanation of travel problems should be given, including jet-lag, hypoxia on flight, diet when overseas and coping with illness while travelling.

For workers in special processes, the role of the nurse may overlap that of the Safety Officer. Both are responsible for promoting safe work procedures and environment, thereby enabling good health and the maximum output of the worker. The nurse may contribute to safety training sessions e.g. by teaching prevention of contact dermatitis. In order to do this she must be fully informed about the risks to health involved in the process carried out. She should also consider workers in those processes where the product is 'at risk' from contamination by the operator, as in domestics in the hospital ward situation, food handling, or preparation of sterile pharmaceuticals. So this group of workers includes not only those who are exposed to specific hazards but also those who could themselves be hazards to the product.

Disabled persons vary from those who are very physically handicapped, to chronic bronchitics. Perhaps the first step in teaching someone how to cope with disability is by association with fellow sufferers. The nurse can therefore encourage membership of specialist societies, e.g. the Multiple Sclerosis Society, where information is assimilated from social gatherings and publications are provided. At the place of work the nurse can encourage the use of prosthesis, diet can be taught for conditions such as diabetes or help given with special toilet facilities where necessary.

Older workers need sensitive, tactful preparation for retirement and understanding of the health changes that may occur. It might be necessary to suggest retraining of pre-retirement staff into less physically exacting work, perhaps in a training or supervisory position, where their experience can be of use to others such as apprentices. The nurse might teach care of the feet, diet and clothing to combat hypothermia and safety in the home. Some companies provide long term pre-retirement courses, covering advice on finances, health, hobbies and coping with loneliness due to loss of work companions. This training is of special value when both husband and wife can attend together, as much more information is retained jointly.

In small companies the nurse may well find herself teaching safety. In matters relating directly to health such as inhalation of dusts or chemical splashes to the skin or eyes, the nurse may have to teach the entire safety committee who will not usually have any medical knowledge. The nurse may be asked to advise on the guarding of machinery or similar problems — she must always seek specialist advice whenever she lacks skilled knowledge, and perhaps arrange for the specialist person to instruct the workers concerned. The nurse might explain the health risks involved when new processes are installed, with the reason for using safety equipment and clothing.

Various legal requirements relate to the training of First Aiders, which will indicate whether the nurse may carry out this teaching herself or should send such staff for training to an approved centre. However, revision instruction will be needed at regular intervals to keep the team in practice, with emphasis on hygiene in general and non-touch technique in cleaning and dressing of wounds in particular. Special treatments relating to the hazards of the process would be taught, such as the care of hydrofluoric acid burns. Procedures to be followed in a major disaster could be practised to ensure efficiency.

Other nursing staff can also benefit from education. The Senior Nursing Officer would be responsible for planning a programme of orientation for new nurses, which might last for two weeks, beginning with attendance at the routine Induction Training held for all new staff. Where only one nurse is employed, adequate time should be allowed for a 'hand over' period in which to train the new nurse. Such a programme would include opportunities to meet the management and to become familiar with the process and its hazards. New nurses might be supervised while carrying out special dressings and procedures such as the use of the Spectrophotometer for estimating blood lead levels, or the carrying out of hearing tests. Where necessary, revision training might be given in nursing procedures such as the treatment of eye injuries. Encouragement to join specialist societies might be given, as nurses learn a great deal from contact with each other. Nurses new to occupational health nursing work can learn much by accompanying a senior nurse on environmental inspections, attendance at safety or other meetings and regularly up-dating her information by reading relevant publications, some of which may be kept in the medical department.

Having decided whom she is going to teach, the nurse must then ask herself the following questions. What is the ethnic and social background of the group? What language problems exist to hinder communication? Will religious background affect acceptance of the subject? What is the average age of the group? Will it be a mixed group of both sexes? Will the group be attending voluntarily or because company policy dictates it? How much prior knowledge does the group have of the subject? All these factors must be considered and assembled as the nurse decides how to approach her students in the group situation. Imagine the situation that would arise, should an over-enthusiastic nurse charge ahead with a lecture on family planning to a group of young, single, Spanish women, perhaps domestics in a hospital or hotel environment. The group would almost certainly be Roman Catholic and such young women having usually been very strictly brought up, the subject itself could be offensive to them; women of Latin origin are very volatile and easily upset, quickly affecting others of the same temperament. This is a hypothetical example but the results of such a situation can be easily imagined!

What Health Topics Should Be Promoted?

Having considered whom she is going to teach, the nurse must then decide what needs exist for education among these groups. Where a Training Manager is employed he should be consulted regarding the selection of subjects to be promoted on a group basis and the programme planned jointly. There may be a company policy giving the basic training responsibilities of the nurse, which she can use as a foundation on which to build.

Health education topics might be related to the process specifically or be general health subjects such as weight control, drug addiction or dental hygiene. The following are just a few suggestions that the nurse might find useful in her programme.

Induction Training, where this is provided, gives the nurse an opportunity to establish health education at the 'source' with all new staff. Such training sessions are intended to familiarise employees with health and safety policies and emergency routines such as fire evacuation, company regulations and staff facilities. Here the nurse may explain her role and the functions of an Occupational Health Service to enable staff to make full use of the facilities provided. She would therefore explain her function regarding treatment, health education, accident prevention, environmental control, health supervision, rehabilitation, counselling, administration, co-operation and records. Following this the nurse might be expected to teach personal hygiene as this is important to all staff. She might teach the care of hair, skin, hands, feet, teeth and include the use of such preparations as deodorants etc., perhaps also mentioning diet briefly. Where Induction Training does not exist in a company, the nurse might approach the Personnel Manager with a request to see all staff on the first day of their appointment and thus establish her education programme.

The nurse may also use hygiene in safety training, relating it to any process where dangerous substances are handled. This would include the teaching of the correct use of 'clean' and 'dirty' washing facilities as in lead processing; the use of hand sinks and monitoring equipment as in areas of possible radioactivity; or the use of barrier or reconditioning creams wherever chemicals are used. In food handling the emphasis would be on cross contamination from septic cuts on fingers, respiratory or gastric infections and strict hygiene. Clothing might be considered as a protection against infection and hazardous substances, but also as a vessel for transmitting such hazards as lead dust or asbestos particles out of the place of work into the home environment, if inadequate care is taken. Control of infection might be explained to hospital maids and porters, who work on wards or the operating theatres. It is not possible to list all the health education topics that apply to the vast number of processes that are carried out but the nurse will discover these for herself as long as she is observant.

Weight control is important to those both over- and underweight. Weight reducing might be taught to those who are simply obese, hypertensive or arthritic and in cardio-vascular disease when it is necessary to reduce the load carried by the feet or to ease strain on the heart. Undernourished persons such as refugees or anorexic young girls might need to be taught correct diet. Weight problems in women are often associated with depressive illness and much encouragement may be needed from the nurse to ensure that the diet is followed. An incentive may be given by the nurse setting a projected goal for her patient to reach within a specified time, monitored by the weekly recording of weight, and where necessary the blood pressure. Competition also stimulates results and this can be provided by forming a group or club of such patients, where the weekly results can be compared and encouragement given.

Dental care is very lacking in many people. Cleaning of teeth after meals should be encouraged, following the correct method, and using the right type of toothbrush. Fluoridation of water, in toothpaste and mouthwashes might be discussed, to prevent gingivitis, periodontitis and pyorrhoea. Fissure sealing of teeth with plastic and ultra-violet light could be explained. Care of false teeth, bone recession and sore gums could be taught with the care of crowned teeth. Regular dental checks should be promoted, along with a diet that provides adequate calcium and omits sweets.

Anti-smoking campaigns are popular as health education subjects, both with nurses and the public. Less people smoke today due to the expense involved and for this reason also many addicted smokers would like to decrease or give up the habit, but do not realise that the solution lies in their own individual determination. The harm done to health by cigarettes could be explained, giving the facts about nicotine yields which vary from 0.3 mg to 1.3 mg per cigarette, the tar yields of 0.7 mg to 12 mg per cigarette and the inhaled smoke which contains carbon monoxide — a chemical asphyxiant. Inhalation of these pollutants is known to exacerbate bronchitis and emphysema and is also thought to cross the placental barrier affecting babies *in utero*, causing them to be smaller. Various anti-smoking devices could be suggested such as chewing gums, tablets and filters which give cigarettes a bitter taste. Again, specialist societies exist to help those who wish to discontinue smoking.

Breast screening is also a significant topic with women, and the teaching of the correct method of breast self-examination is important, using the palms of the hands rather than the fingertips. This procedure is important after the birth of children and during the menopause and should ideally be carried out at the end of each menstrual period. In some large companies and hospitals consideration has been given to providing mammography for female staff, but this is very expensive. Cervical cytology could also be promoted, provided that a Medical Officer is available to carry out a proper pelvic examination or, failing this, a mobile unit with specially trained staff could be asked to visit the place of work — which again is expensive.

Drug addiction is an increasing problem of modern day society, affecting mainly young people; using both hard drugs (opiates, cocaine, etc.) and soft drugs (cannabis, barbiturates etc.) The increasing doses needed with greater tolerance, with the resulting moral, physical and mental deterioration, could be explained. The risk of hepatitis and septicaemia from unsterile intravenous injections (mainlining), the birth of addicted babies and poor life expectancy could be discussed. Sources of help might be given in such a way that those needing assistance need not have to identify themselves in order to obtain help, but can be assured that the nurse will advise them if asked. Again specialist societies and hospital clinics exist to help drug addicts.

Foot care is greatly needed by anyone engaged in jobs that require constant standing or walking; correct shoes suitable to the process involved might be the first basis for education. Such shoes might include re-inforced toecaps, flat rubber soles and uppers made of leather to allow the circulation of air. Measurement of feet to ensure a proper fit is important and allowance should be made for the wearing of inner soles or hosettes to absorb excess perspiration. Chiropody treatment could be promoted for diabetics and older staff in particular but for anyone with corns and hard skin in general. The control of varicose veins using elastic stockings and elevating the legs to encourage venous return from the lower limbs, might be taught. The results of neglecting varicose veins, namely the manifestation of eczema which breaks down into ulcers could be explained. Exercise and weight are important and in pregnancy support hose may be needed if there is aching or swelling of the legs.

Other topics that might be promoted could include contraception, care of the eyes, hearing conservation, specific hazards related to the process, lifting techniques, alcohol abuse and food handling. The nurse needs to look at the process and the working environment to assess the needs for education, by identifying job hazards and areas where knowledge is lacking in health matters.

When Should Health Be Promoted?

Group education may be formal by arrangement with the management or it may be spontaneous occurring during meetings or environmental inspections. Formal group education may be required at specified intervals for particular staff, on particular subjects, as a matter of policy. Such expectations might only exist where a Training Manager is responsible for implementing a programme within given specifications. Records would be kept by him of all formal group training carried out by the nurse and she would be expected to consult with him when formulating projected health education programmes, for which expenditure must be allocated.

Spontaneous group education might occur at meetings of the safety committee or perhaps line management. The nurse could be asked to explain the health hazards of a new process, or the risk of infection from an illness among the staff, e.g. tuberculosis, or explain the benefits of a special programme to be carried out, such as influenza innoculations.

The time, place and environment for group training should be chosen with care. At the end of a busy shift the employees will not be as alert as when rested and if they are piece-workers they will not appreciate being removed from work unless they are paid while attending for training. The environment and place chosen should be conducive to learning, a quiet location with good lighting and ventilation and comfortable seating. Distractions such as telephones, traffic or machinery should be avoided. Individual education is generally spontaneous and takes place between the nurse and an employee in a variety of circumstances, some of which are described below.

The pre-employment health interview is an ideal situation for the nurse to start teaching health, either from observations made of the applicant's physical state or from the preventive health and safety aspect of the job for which he has applied.

The treatment situation gives a further opportunity to teach. The cause of an accident might be explored and safety principles mentioned. Staff who regularly report with the same problem which could be controlled with help, can be seen as in need of education. This might apply to recurrent cases of skin irritation, insomnia, etc.

Individual education might also be given during environmental inspections carried out by the nurse. Here it might be necessary to demonstrate a correct lifting technique or to promote the safe storage of inflammable or other dangerous chemicals. Or, the nurse may request to see an individual after an inspection if she considers it more tactful to see him alone, as when the person concerned is of management or supervisory grading. He would otherwise be embarrassed by the nurse, in front of the men whom he controls.

Education, in fact, occurs every day in normal conversations between the nurse and other members of staff, as when enquiring about someone's progress after illness, about a wife who is away on maternity leave or about a child in hospital. It also includes discussions about routine daily occurrences such as the installation of a new process or plant. In fact, unless the nurse is careful, she may well find that all conversations over lunch centre around health topics!

Individual teaching may be arranged at the request of a departmental head, perhaps because a need exists for a talk on personal hygiene, or because of persistent absences from work — possibly due either to the individual's health or a domestic problem. Poor sleeping habits and, therefore, an inability to wake up on time, may be the cause of bad time-keeping.

An employee may ask to see the nurse for advice on problems related to his wife or children. In particular, parents of young children frequently turn to the company nurse for advice on feeding problems, babies that do not sleep properly or older children with infectious illness. Care of elderly relatives is also a frequent cause for the nurse's advice to be sought. Additionally a head of department may ask to see the nurse for discussion on the management of an ill employee who is on restricted work.

The counselling situation can also be used if a need is seen by the nurse for health instruction. However, as counselling is not intended for this purpose the nurse must be careful not to loose sight of her role as a counsellor.

How Can Health Education Be Carried Out?

Various forms of teaching can be used, which include the spoken and written word, visual learning and practical learning.

The Spoken Word

(a) Group discussion is carried out in a comfortable situation, with the group seated, all able to hear and see each other. Everyone contributes to the discussion, without any one person monopolising the conversation, which should be concentrated in one direction.

(b) Syndicate discussion is the method by which the group is broken up into several smaller groups who disperse for discussion on a set subject, for a set period of time. At the end of the time the groups return to report back.

(c) Plenary discussion is the group discussion which follows a syndicate recess. At this the findings and conclusions from the syndicate discussions are explored by the whole group.

(d) Case discussions are when one particular case, topic, problem or item is discussed at length.

(e) Buzz groups are used to encourage audiences to relax, or to stimulate interest. Each person is asked to talk briefly to the person next to him for a few minutes, usually before question time, or to provide a break in a long lecture.

(f) A symposium is the discussion of a topic by several speakers without audience participation.

(g) A seminar is when a number of papers to the same topic are given followed by audience participation.

(h) A lecture is a prepared talk given without interruption.

(i) The Socratic method of teaching is used when the teacher questions the class with skill in order to make the class think out the subject for themselves.

The Written Word

This includes individual research as in the writing of specific projects, test papers and reports; it also includes the reading of journals, publications and hand-out material following instruction. It would apply to individual notes about visits made for observation purposes, notes taken during lectures or notes for reference. Literature such as a company's Health and Safety Policy, staff manual or written procedures to be followed in emergency would also be included, as would correspondence with various organisations which provide information on request to the public.

Visual Education

This includes visits to exhibitions and working situations for observation purposes; the use of mechanical aids such as films, slides, the over-head projector, television, flannelgraph and the chalk board. The use of items such as artificial wounds which adhere to the skin, or the use of the skeleton in First Aid training, could be mentioned here. Demonstration teaching is included, when special techniques are shown, such as different methods of lifting or use of stretchers. Role play might be used, when students act out a situation before an audience for discussion later. Visual training also includes specific campaigns carried out using permanent displays in the medical and training departments, the subjects of which would be rotated or changed at regular intervals. Such a display might consist of wall mounted notice boards situated in corridors, lifts or large staff areas. Free-standing display units or showcases could also be used. In this way posters, brochures, photographs and actual articles could be displayed, arranged to contrast attractively and capture attention.

In large areas, such as a long corridor, the display might conform to one theme; in small areas the subject should be applicable to the work done — such as the safe storage of explosive substances in workshops, or food hygiene in staff canteens. In safety displays the actual items that have caused injury might be shown, items such as exploded aerosol cannisters, defective gloves and sharp instruments. Where a photography department exists, as in hospitals or companies with Press Offices, pictures might be taken of hazardous situations and a display made. It is important that all displays should be colourful, well planned and that individual items should contrast and be displayed clearly and neatly. Lettering should be clear and large enough to be read easily.

Practical Teaching

This is the method used when students learn by 'doing' the procedure under discussion. This could mean the carrying out of special tests in the medical department by new nurses, under supervision, or learning by accompanying a senior nurse on environmental inspections. This is also known as 'Actuality Learning'. Practical teaching may also be used in a simulated training environment and would apply to the training of First Aiders using a Resusci-Anne manikin, on which cardiac massage and artificial respirations are taught. It would also apply to the teaching of non-touch techniques in would dressing, using the facility of the medical department. This is known as 'Simulation Learning'.

Personal Example

This is another form of teaching — the nurse is constantly watched by the employees and she must be seen to do as she teaches. Her appearance should be spotless and her uniform complete — thus she illustrates her teaching on hygiene and in the wearing of her uniform represents her profession. When in hazardous areas she should wear the correct protective clothing and be seen to use safety equipment where applicable. Nurses cannot, for instance, insist that catering staff should wear protective headwear if the nurse herself does not wear a protective cap when she inspects food handling or food storage areas! Within the medical department also, the example of the senior nurse will be noted and copied, not only in the wearing of uniforms but also in unsafe practices. An example of this might be the omission on the part of the nurse to wear actinotherapy goggles herself, when administering ultra-violet light to a patient — however well she has protected her patient.

Planning a Health Education Session

Having decided whom she is going to teach, what her subject will be, when and in what form it will be done, the nurse must now decide how to present her session. For this she must first allow herself sufficient time to ensure that she is adequately prepared to give such training, and able to answer any questions that may arise, from her students. She must, therefore, research her subject thoroughly and prepare a teaching plan for her own guidance while teaching. This plan should be divided into two sections, one for the teaching outline, the other for practical details to be remembered. For this a double page of foolscap paper can be used, as is shown in Table 6.1. By way of an example, let us construct a plan for Induction Training, applicable to every company that employs occupational health nurses. The page relating to the subject matter should be laid out in a series of logical steps as follows:

1. Class Composition

This should include the number of students expected, the average age of the group, the extent of their prior knowledge of the subject and, where applicable, the nationality of the majority — should a language problem exist.

2. The Time Allowed

This should include sufficient time for questions from the group, in the concluding stage.

3. The Subject

The name of the session i.e. The function of the Occupational Health Service.

Table 6.1: Teaching Plan

Practical Details	Subject Matter
1. Method	1. Class composition
2. Seating	2. Time allowed
3. Equipment	3. Subject
4. Difficult words	4. Topic
5. Visual aids	5. Aims
6. Timing	6. Objectives
7. Hand-out material	7. Introduction in full
	Logical steps 1.
	2.
	3.
	4.
	5.
	8. Conclusion

4. Topic

This is the particular item for discussion i.e. the specific company's Occupational Health Service.

5. Aim

This is what the nurse wishes to achieve by her lecture, i.e. to familiarise new staff with services and facilities available.

6. Object

This is the result required from the information passed on by the nurse, i.e. to enable staff to make full use of the service.

7. Introduction

The opening sentence should be written out in full and it is always useful to begin with a definition of the subject to be covered, i.e. Occupational Health. This would then be expanded into logical steps, perhaps using the ten basic functions as an outline and relating each to the individual company's policy or operation, as follows:

(a)	Treatment	(b)	Health Education
(c)	Environmental Control	(d)	Health Supervision
(e)	Counselling	(f)	Accident Prevention
(g)	Rehabilitation	(h)	Administration

    (i)   Co-operation   (j)   Records

8. Conclusion

A brief resume of the key points should be made by the instructor and she should confirm that the teaching has been assimilated either by asking direct questions of the individual student, or asking 'open' questions not directed at any particular student. Questions from them should also be encouraged. Hand-out material may then be given out; it is not advisable to issue this earlier, unless it is needed for reference during the class, as attention will be distracted from the instructor.

The page relating to the practical details should also be laid out in logical steps as follows:

1. Method

This is the type of teaching session, e.g. lecture, demonstration or discussion etc., and should include the amount of class activitiy involved.

2. Seating

This will depend on the method chosen. For demonstration sessions, the furniture would be arranged in a semi-circle in front of the instructor and her equipment, with space allowed, if needed, for group participation. For discussion, seating would be either in a circle or around a table. It is important that students are seated close enough to hear the speaker and to see visual aids. The speaker must also decide what position she will adopt when teaching; in order to be heard at the back of the room it might be necessary to stand, unless she is on a platform; or a microphone might be supplied if the venue is a conference hall.

3. Equipment

All equipment that will be needed should be listed in order of use. Items such as spare or coloured chalk should be included.

4. Difficult words

Long or difficult words should be printed clearly in case they have to be written up on the chalk board. Short quotations may be written out in full or reference material should be ready with the passage clearly marked.

5. Visual aids

Note should be made when the different aids are to be used during the class.

6. Timing

It is useful to note at different stages how much time should have elapsed, and to check this against a clock which should be visible at the back of the room, as the class progresses.

7. Hand-out material

This should be listed, to be given out at the end of the class.

Having prepared her teaching plan and researched her subject thoroughly, the nurse must always check that the arrangements requested for her teaching session have been completed. Using her plan, all equipment should be checked to ensure that everything is in working order — such as the correct plugs to match the electrical sockets, that seating is correctly arranged and equipment such as chalk boards are provided and are clean.

No teaching session should be without visual aids, as these hold the attention. There are many kinds of visual aids, which can either be bought via a Training Department, borrowed from various sources (discussed in the section on sources of help) or the nurse might improvise her own with a little imagination. Some useful equipment which the nurse might find helpful in her teaching programme is described below.

Chalk boards are now available in both green and black background with metal backing. On these, coloured chalks may be used or magnetic aids can be placed and re-arranged as desired on the surface. These aids might be figures, words or outlines of objects — anything that might be useful. Chalk boards, when free-standing on easels, may also be supplied with one side covered with flannelette. To this aids may be attached, if also made of flannelette, but paper aids may also be used if a strip of sandpaper is stuck to the back of each. In this way, cut out figures or pictures can be applied to the flannelette covered board by applying a slight pressure against the sandpaper. 'Prick' drawings can also be used on the chalk board — this is when the outline of a drawing is put on the board using faint dots only and these are drawn in properly when needed during the class. When using the chalk board the nurse must plan ahead and allow adequate space for the subject matter that she intends to put up.

Slides and films should be viewed before being shown, ensuring that both the projector screen and lens are clean and free of dead insects or dust particles, which will distract from the film itself. The over-head projector is another very useful item of equipment; here the slides should be stacked in order of use before the class begins and the focus checked. Flip charts may be used, either for a sequence of large drawings, or for showing calculations etc. Again all lettering should be clear and as much colour as possible be used. The episcope projects a diagram from paper onto the chosen background, e.g. a chalk board, and the silhouette is then drawn in, perhaps using dots only, until needed.

After giving her lecture, the nurse may be required to complete a report for the Training Manager, stating who attended the class, what the subject was and for how long the session lasted. It is also useful to ask the Manager to find out if the students found the class beneficial, in order that faults may be rectified, or improvements suggested. In the absence of a Training Manager the nurse might still keep records of the teaching done by herself, as this information is useful when she wants permission for expenditure on films or equipment. A specimen of a suitable training report form is shown in Table 6.2, as a guide to such record keeping. Such records would apply only to the formal group teaching done, as most individual education would take place on a confidential basis, as in the treatment situation.

Table 6.2: Training Record

Location_____					Date_____		
Employee/Trainee			Training Completed				Instructor
Name and initials	Job Title	Clock Number	Title or description of training	Type of training	Location of training	Time	Names and initials

Sources of Help in Health Education

Nurses are not usually adequately prepared during their general training for their role as educators in health. Some training in teaching is therefore necessary before this function can be carried out efficiently.

Occupational health nurses can seek this instruction from three sources, beginning with their own company or organisation. Most Industrial Training Boards run two week courses, for employees within the specified industries, to train as Registered Instructors. Some companies provide their own Instructor's Certificates, with the Training Board's approval. The nurse could begin, therefore, by approaching her management to enquire about such courses.

Where an industry does not provide Instructor's Courses, the nurse could apply to the Health Education Council who run Health Education Certificate Courses at various technical colleges. These courses may be day-release or block courses and charge a fee, and application should be made to the local Area Health Authority. Special courses are also provided for the Audio-Visual Officers Certificate, which deals mainly in the use of mechanical visual aids.

The Royal College of Nursing, London, provides intensive training in teaching methods, as part of the Occupational Health Nurse Certificate Course and in short courses. Application should be made to the Director of Education, Royal College of Nursing.

For nurses not able to train in the near future, but who are anxious to start a health education programme, the local Health Education Department will plan a programme to specification on request. They will give any assistance, including the provision of equipment, films, leaflets etc., but will not actually carry out the teaching itself.

The British Red Cross and St John's Ambulance Association will also lend equipment such as Resusci-Anne manikins and First Aid films, and will provide speakers for a fee. The British Safety Council runs various safety courses, but will also provide speakers, again for a fee, on specific safety topics such as kinetic lifting, legislation etc. The local Environmental Health Inspectors will speak free of charge on food handling and legislation, providing films and literature. This practice varies with different boroughs.

The Pre-Retirement Association runs courses at the place of work for staff due to retire. Subjects covered include health and safety, finances, leisure interests, living arrangements and coping with loneliness due to loss of work companions. One day seminars are run for up to seven couples, or fourteen individuals. Additionally, three day courses are run for a maximum of sixty people. Both husband and wife are asked to attend together, as more is learnt in this way.

The Family Planning Association also provides one day courses, either in contraception or in psychosexual problems. Application should be made to the Education Unit, Family Planning Association, Mortimer Street, London, W1, and not to the local branches of the Association.

Various films are available from different film libraries and audio-visual centres; some companies who produce pharmaceuticals, e.g. influenza innoculations, will also lend films or carry out a 'presentation' providing that a sale is assured by the company concerned.

Nearly all specialist societies, such as the British Diabetic Association, Multiple Sclerosis Society or the Mastectomy Association will provide individual literature on request for specific staff.

There are many sources of help available to occupational health nurses in carrying out their role in health education. Those mentioned are but a very few and as nurses identify new needs for education they will also find new sources of information by enquiry and by research.

Further Reading

R. Borger and A. Seaborne, *The Psychology of Learning* (Penguin, Middlesex, 1970)

A. Burkitt, 'What is Health Education?', *Nursing Times* (23 June 1977), pp.3, 5, 7

E. Ensins, 'How and When: Practical Aspects of Health Education in Hospitals', *Royal Society of Health*, vol.4 (1974) pp.183-5

Health Education Journal (Health Education Council, London)

H.R. Mills, *Teaching and Training* (Macmillan, London, 1972)

J. Monks, 'Economical Slide-making', *Nursing Times* (17 August 1978), p.381

L. Powell, *Communication and Learning* (Pitman, London, 1973)

H. Runswick and C. Davis, *Health Education – Practical Teaching Techniques* (HM & M Publishers, Aylesbury, 1975)

G.J. Russell, *Teaching in Further Education* (Pitman, London, 1972)

'Training in Health Education', *Occupational Health*, vol.27, no.11 (November 1975), pp.496-7

7 COUNSELLING

Frances Baker

Listen to me, do but listen,
and let that be the comfort you offer me.
Bear with me while I have my say;
When I have finished you may mock.
May not I too voice my thoughts.   Job 21.

These words from the Old Testament, written so many years ago, are probably as pertinent today as they were then. Life is full of hustle, time is precious and the prospect of spending it silently while another person speaks does not, for many of us, have much appeal. In addition, nurses are people of action; we pride ourselves on the amount of activity we can crowd into an hour, the immeasurable difficulties we can surmount. Listening, in comparison, seems a somewhat flat activity. Yet the Oxford Dictionary definition of the word implies a rather different emphasis, for the word listen is defined as 'to make an effort to hear something, hear a person speaking with attention'. To listen, then, is an active rather than a passive state, and the one who participates is playing a definite role rather than merely being present. To know how to listen requires the ability to attend, both physically and psychologically; to be in a state of readiness to absorb all the sounds and signs that follow and then respond to the behaviour, feelings and the meaning behind the speaker's comments.

Counselling is thus a formal development of listening. It has been variously described as a process of interaction, usually and hopefully therapeutic in intention and outcome, between two people – the counsellor and the client. At the conclusion the client will have reached a decision on some matter of personal concern by verbally working through its varying facets. The emphasis for action is thus firmly on the part of the client, not the counsellor, whose principal contribution is that of enabler – allowing or assisting the other to achieve his purpose.

Before enlarging on a definition of counselling, its techniques, organisation and pitfalls, it would seem appropriate to devote some space to considering whatever implications there are for the practice of occupational health nursing, and whether in fact such nurses should be acting as 'counsellors'. Perhaps a good starting point would be to relate an incident which occurred at a recent British Institute of Management series of workshops[1] on the subject of 'Stress in Industry'. The final session was devoted to a question and answer period with a consultant psychiatrist as one of the panel of experts. A manager from the audience asked what immediate step he might take to cope with and prevent any stress in his organisation. The psychiatrist quickly replied 'Get yourself a well trained occupational health nurse!'

Those who feel that this cap fits are no doubt nodding sagely at his words and feeling quietly proud, and rightly so. Yet consider for a moment the implication of his words and the context in which they were expressed. If one were to ask a group of student nurses what an occupational health nurse is, the reply would most surely be, 'A nurse who works in industry'. To some extent this is of course true, for many of them do, although not all. The description is far from accurate, however, for there has been no emphasis on the word 'health'. An occupational health nurse is one whose work is concerned with the relationship between the job which a person does and his health, health in this context following the description of WHO/ILO[2] as 'a balance between three states, physical, mental and social', or, as some would express it, body, mind and spirit. When the balance is upset, when disharmony arises, when undue stress is placed in any of these areas, then disease may result. The causes of physical stress are fairly easily recognised by any nurse who knows the way her organisation works, be it long hours, unduly heavy labour, bad conditions, or a host of other factors which a routine environmental survey would reveal. The results of physical stress are not over long in revealing themselves, and the right kind of pressure exerted in the right places ought to bring results sooner or later. Mental and social stress, however, are more difficult to appreciate, nor do they seem as serious in comparison with the physical — in the initial phase as least. Yet, increasingly, medical science is coming to recognise that man is a total being and that the disease which presents physically may be mental or social in origin. Such conditions, moreover, are often more difficult to resolve than those whose causes are straightforward and physical.

Given this recognition, prevention is all important and by the very nature of her position, the contribution of the occupational health nurse is crucial if any measure of success is to be achieved. Occupational health nurses are almost the only health care practitioners whose routine work takes them into contact with the 'healthy' adult population of this country. Thus, if the disease causation theory described above is even partially accurate, then the preventive role of the occupational health practitioner is clearly of vital importance. Equally, by the very nature of the occupational health role, such nurses ought to find it easier to assume the mantle of counsellor than would nurses from other branches of the profession, who are more normally associated with the sick, the young and the aged, and whose role is a more naturally directive one.

While members of the work force will present themselves at the surgery as patients as the need arises, there will be lengthy periods when they will not require the nurse's professional ministrations. The nurse will then be the man or woman to whom they chat over lunch in the canteen, about cars, or holidays, or the trials of coping with their respective teenager's current vagaries. He will be the hero who scored the vital goal in the football match. She will be one who, to everybody's amusement, pulled a muscle running to stop a ball for the ladies' cricket team. The natural role may be as friend and colleague as well as nurse.

This situation is one of the joys and potential sorrows of working in industry, as opposed to a hospital. The joys lie in that one finds oneself making many friends at all levels of the work force who give strength and enrichment to one's own life. The abstract qualities that most readily spring to mind from my personal recollections of life as a nurse at a colliery are wisdom and humour. On reflection, there were at least as many lessons of life to be learned in that rather grimy situation as I absorbed during my training years in a leading Scottish teaching hospital. As already indicated though, sorrows too are an equal concomitant. When a fatal accident or sudden death occurs, the victim is not the stranger who suddenly arrives in a casualty department or the intensive care unit. He is the pit deputy with whom you joked an hour previously, when he came to the medical centre on some routine matter; he is the young electrician who confided that he was about to get engaged to be married. The caring manner but professional detachment which the hospital nurse acquires as a necessary safeguard to her emotions is not so readily available to the occupational health nurse. Even the experienced nurse working in industry still finds such happenings traumatic for her own emotions.

Working in a heavy industry such as mining or steel making, the fatal accident is always there as a potential threat; one might say accidents, because of the almost uncanny way in which serious accidents never seem to happen singly. The dead or seriously injured worker is or has been part of the group of which the nurse is a member. The maturity of understanding which results from living through such experiences has much to do with creating the kind of background which contributes in no small measure to becoming 'a good occupational health nurse' and a potentially successful counsellor, in a way in which no amount of abstract reading on the subject can do.

There is a sense, too, in which the nurse working in a light industry, where the threat of death is a less obviously constant companion, has a slightly different but no less real problem. Cardiovascular accidents tend to be no respecters of time or place and are as likely, if not more so, to occur at the place of work. This 'bolt from the blue' type of happening can be even more upsetting than the one which takes place in an industry where it is an ever present possibility. Because of the close relationship, which the occupational health nurse has with people in the organisation, it is much easier for her to see those who present in the counselling situation as clients rather than patients. The difference may appear slight but it is much more than merely quibbling semantics. The role which each plays is subtly but critically different. The word 'patient', derived as it is from the Latin word for suffering, indicates a state where things happen to one; it is a passive state and thus one of relative inactivity. A client, however, is a much more active participant in a situation and the relationship between client and counsellor is very different from that which exists between nurse and patient, even though in the industrial setting the same characters may participate as client or patient in different circumstances.

So far it has been suggested that there is a relationship between stress and ill-health in the widest sense of the word, that the occupational health nurse has a vital preventive part to play and that the counselling situation is the appropriate medium for what will hopefully be therapeutic action. Among nurses working in industry varying degrees of expertise are normally found, so that while one has the ability to readily absorb the complexities of toxicology, another will have an excellent grasp of legislation, whilst a third will be particularly adept at applying the kind of dressing that stays secure throughout the most strenuous working shift. Nevertheless, each will have to apply herself to acquiring the various skills. Equally, although some nurses are good listeners, the basic requirement in counselling, others will need to make a conscious effort in this direction. The practice of counselling, however, consists in more than simply listening and, although much of it is an art, there is a considerable body of observed and recorded knowledge on the subject that can be learned.

The act of counselling has already been briefly described, but a fuller description is that found in the report of the Steering Committee of the

Standing Conference for the Advancement of Counselling 1969:[3]

> Counselling is a process through which one person helps another by
> purposeful conversation in an understanding atmosphere. It seeks to
> establish a helping relationship in which the one counsellor can
> express his thoughts and feelings in such a way as to clarify his own
> situation, come to terms with some new experience, see his difficulty
> more objectively, and so face his problem with less anxiety and
> tension. The basic purpose is to assist the individual to make his own
> decision from among the choices open to him.

Those who are involved in this situation are usually only the counsellor
(in the present context the occupational health nurse) and the client.
The client is obviously a person seeking help with a problem although,
again in the occupational health context, it may be related to a nurse/
patient meeting. For instance, we have all met the worker who presents
one or more times with a fairly trivial injury or illness before he gets
round to the real problem that is worrying him. In this kind of situation
it may well be that the nurse will consciously have to change from the
more authoritarian attitude of nurse to the receptive one of counsellor,
depending on the nature of the problem. If all that is required is medical
information on some other physical sign or symptom, then of course,
no change of role is required. Problems, in the counselling sense, are
rather different. Here there is a difficulty of some kind where a solution
is not so readily available and where the details may be complex and
require considerable unravelling. Indeed, what at first may appear a
fairly simple matter can, on further elucidation, assume gigantic
proportions.

Nevertheless, decisions as to the action required must come from the
client, not the counsellor. Certainly, if factual information is required,
then this ought to be given, e.g. in the case of an unmarried pregnant
worker the nurse ought to know not just the names of the various
statutory and non-statutory bodies who can provide help but their
exact location in the area, times when they are open, appointment
systems and so on. But the ultimate decisions must be made by the girl
herself. The function of the nurse is that of enabler, i.e. 'to supply a
person with the means to do something' (Oxford Dictionary). In the
example cited, there are several possible courses of action, the
implications of each of which require calm consideration before the
client makes up her mind. The nurse/counsellor's part is so to conduct
her side of the partnership that the client is in no doubt that her own

views and emotions are both recognised and accepted. An atmosphere of trust must be present and the client helped to recognise what are her innermost feelings on her problem. This is done in part by the nurse appreciating what the girl is saying, and then reflecting this back to her with more exact meaning. Thus, the girl can recognise for herself the feelings and emotions which may previously have been present largely in her subconscious mind. Feelings and drives that have hitherto been hidden have a chance to come to the surface and be clarified, either by the counsellor acting as a sound board or, in more complex situations, through a measure of positive assistance.

It will be clear already from what has been said that just as listening implies more than simply being silent while someone else is speaking, so counselling is a much more complex relationship than perhaps it appears at first sight. Listening means actively absorbing what is being said, counselling uses this tool on the material of knowledge. Any occupational health nurse worthy of the name knows her work place — what the hazards are, how the various processes take place etc., but the knowledge required for counselling is more than this. The nurse must be able to enter, in an abstract sense at least, the client's world, whether he comes from shop floor or management. The purpose of this is to know what are his values, what he feels about work, what kind of social life he has and what kind of culture he comes from, in order that the help that is given be both relevant and constructive.

A tall order, indeed, and one which only becomes possible by the extent to which the counsellor understands herself. Self knowledge, the ability to accept and understand oneself, is essential if one is to be of any real assistance to others. From this follows the sensitivity and openness towards others which helps them to solve their problems through the growth of their personalities. It would be false advice, however, to suggest that all problems are capable of solution. Fairy stories have various settings and tell many different tales, yet there are certain characteristics which they have in common, one of which is the happy ending. Unfortunately, real life is often rather different and problems do not always go away. A measure of Shakespeare's greatness is his understanding of many of life's underlying tragedies and his ability to express them. *King Lear* ends with these words:

The weight of this sad time we must obey;
Speak what we feel, not what we ought to say.
The oldest hath borne most: we that are young,
Shall never see so much nor live so long.

The complex plot and sub-plots have been resolved, but the ending is quiet acceptance and hope for the future, not wedding bells and a fanfare of trumpets. Likewise, it may well be that the problem is one with which the client will have to learn to live and adjust his life accordingly. An extreme example of such a situation would be the young man confined to a wheelchair following àn accident at work. No amount of counselling skill is going to bring back full mobility to someone who is paraplegic and it would be cruel to pretend otherwise. Factual information is of course useful; it helps to know what benefits are available to someone in this position, what kind of personal problems, physical, mental and social may already be present or be a future possibility: but the most important requirement is empathy — 'the power of projecting one's personality into (and so fully comprehending) the object of contemplation' (Oxford Dictionary) — in other words, feeling something of what the other is experiencing. This does not mean, however, saying to the paraplegic, 'I know what it's like, I once broke my leg and couldn't get around for ages'. No one, unless they too have permanently lost the use of their legs can possibly understand what such a person is enduring. Those who are disabled are very quick to recognise the difference. The nurse who has suffered bereavement, who has a problem child, an elderly dependant relative or some other ongoing problem and has coped more or less successfully with it, ought to have a head start on those whom the difficulties of living have hardly touched. It is 'being with' the client in spirit without perhaps very much actually being said. The right kind of silence often says much more than any amount of trite phrases can achieve.

Counselling, however, need not be confined to the crisis situations such as those to which reference has already been made — the pregnant single girl and the disabled worker. Assistance with the resolution of problems is its most accepted province but if this is the extent of responsibility then the role must needs be a very limited one, confined as it will be to making the best of a bad job. It is a situation similar to that which sees the occupational health nurse as a sticker on of plasters and a giver out of aspirin. Counselling could and should have a preventive side so that people could be assisted to anticipate problems through help and training until they reach the kind of maturity whereby they can act as their own counsellors.

Any counselling, if properly conducted, ought to result in development of the client's personality, but if the experience is confined to a single flash point situation then the extent of growth is likely to be limited. A medical model to demonstrate this premise might be the way in which peptic ulcers are treated, e.g., tension → pain → antacid → relief → tension → pain → etc. While another approach could be: tension → pain → antacid → conscious practised relaxation — and hopefully, in time, a diminution of the features which caused the problem in the first place. This is perhaps to oversimplify the problem, as any ulcer sufferer would be quick to point out, but the principle is a legitimate one and at least worthy of consideration.

This is not to ignore the fact that there can be a therapeutic result from a crisis situation. As those who are experienced in the area of psychiatry will know, there is a school which maintains that at the height of a crisis there is a moment when, because of and in the midst of the momentum, a transforming change can begin in one who is mentally ill. Crisis Intervention, as this approach is termed, has many advocates, but it is a highly specialised kind of treatment and obviously unsuitable for an occupational health centre, besides which the severely mentally ill person is hardly likely to be at work! The growth of personality that is being sought is synonymous with all that is appropriate to preventive medicine and, consequently, an area where the occupational health nurse could have an important role.

Within the work situation, problems are likely to arise in a variety of identifiable areas. They may be personal to an individual or they may result from a situation within the framework of the place or associated with the work process, or yet again, from extraneous matters which may or may not be having repercussions on the work of an individual. These problems can exist separately but are equally likely to overlap, for it is a very strong personality indeed which can divorce one aspect of life when forced to deal with another. Individual problems are obviously legion, but there are certain broad categories which tend to encompass a multiplicity of common factors.

Before looking further at the areas where difficulties arise it would perhaps be helpful to consider the importance of basic human needs, for so often it is because of the failure to take these into account that problems present themselves in the first place. The definitive work on the subject has been done by A.H. Maslow,[4] who categorised needs as follows:

Physiological	— food, drink, air, warmth, sleep, shelter, sex, excretion.
Social	— sense of belonging. Giving and receiving of friendship and love. Social activities.
Egotistical	— self respect and the respect of others. Autonomy

and responsibility, appreciation and recognition.
Achievement, knowledge, status.

Psychological — growth and personal development.
Accomplishments and talents fully used.
Creativity.

Needs in the work setting have been further described by Herzberg *et al.*[5] as being in two broad areas which are worthy of consideration if dissatisfaction is to be avoided and satisfaction stimulated. The first of these areas is related to bodily comforts and covers such factors as space, heating, lighting and other general facilities such as canteens, break times, sanitary and washing facilities. The second category is concerned with motivation and responsibility. The importance of each or both of these needs will obviously vary for different individuals for various reasons at differing periods. The needs of the young unmarried man are likely to be quite opposite to those of the working mother. The man nearing retirement thinks very differently from the one with a young family and his place still to establish.

The contrast has to be appreciated if constructive assistance is to be given. If basic needs are not met then a sense of insecurity is produced and other problems tend to follow. An example might be a case where a miner in the fifties age group, suffering from a significant percentage of pneumoconiosis and living in an area of high unemployment, learns that his pit is likely to close. The problem here is likely to be psychological as much as financial but much will depend on the personality of the man in question and his particular social needs.

It is, however, within the framework of the work situation that most difficulties arise. It is not easy to define the point at which a social/psychological problem becomes potentially hazardous to health. Measurement of the extent of the problem is equally difficult, which is perhaps one of the reasons why, when the question of Health and Safety arises, emphasis is placed on the latter part. Safety, or, perhaps more accurately, the lack of it, is easily recognised, and the results can be tabulated, made into statistics and analysed endlessly. Health is a much more nebulous area where, although no one would dispute its worth, few would feel prepared to argue its cost effectiveness. If a man receives a laceration sufficient to keep him away from work then the matter is quite straightforward — cleanse, dress, record, investigate, follow up. Casual absenteeism, however, which may well have stress of some kind as a root cause, is less easily identifiable. In addition, such evidence as exists seems to show that short-period sickness absence is on the increase whereas accident rates in many industries appear to be dropping.

The nurse, particularly by observing and listening when outside the surgery, has the opportunity to notice the kind of work on which individuals are engaged, the pressure under which they are working, or, conversely, the monotony of certain tasks. For some people the fact that their skills are being under-used can be as stressful as a position where the work is too heavy or demanding mentally or physically.

People in authority who lack good leadership qualities can make life very difficult for those under them. The manager who rules in a heavy handed manner, or who delegates to the point of abdication, can equally cause symptoms of stress in the work force, likewise the type who never seems to know his mind from one week to the next. Similarly, the manager may feel that he does not get the co-operation to which he is entitled, that his colleagues are trying to undermine his authority and, in fact, that everyone is against him.

In his book *Future Shock*[6] Alvin Toffler has shown that the amount of change which an individual experiences has a cumulative effect on him both psychologically, as one might expect, but also physiologically. The kind of change which he studied included movement from one job or place to another at fairly short intervals of time, although the motivation is also worthy of consideration. Miners from Eastern Europe, fleeing from their homeland, appeared to have fewer settling-in problems than did colliers forced by pit closures to move from the North of England to the Midlands. Other situation changes noted by Toffler which produce effects include the following: movement into a different culture, particularly if this is to another country with major differences in social customs and attitudes; rapid turnover among colleagues, subordinates or bosses; frequent changes in job objectives or standards of performance. The nature and structure of industry today suggests that this tendency will increase rather than lessen in the future.

Problems which have their origin outside the organisation and appear to be unrelated to the work situation may not at first sight appear to come within the province of the occupational health nurse. However, if one accepts the view of man as the sum of all his experiences, then that which takes place outside the working environment cannot be excluded from consideration. The types of problem of this kind are legion and in some degree or other are shared by most people. A list might consist of the following examples: money — or more particularly the lack of it; the way in which husbands and wives arrange their joint finances, and indeed the whole gamut of marital relations and associated problems; the way in which children behave; problems with parents and other relatives; sex difficulties, both heterosexual and homosexual; addictions, whether to alcohol, drugs or smoking and problems within the family, from educational difficulties at one end to the elderly invalid at the other. The range of problems gives added emphasis to the need for the counselling occupational health nurse to have as wide a spectrum of useful knowledge and information at her finger tips as possible.

Availability of counselling support at the time of need is important. If someone with a problem has perhaps summoned up the courage to come and talk to the nurse then it can be quite disastrous if no one is there. This obviously presents difficulties in a single nurse establishment but need not invariably do so if a pattern of availability is well publicised – when the nurse is in the surgery, when around the works, when not on duty, etc. People with problems are often so wrapped up in their particular difficulty, understandably so, that they can sometimes be very lacking in patience. Others, however, with seemingly overwhelming odds against them, have an almost saint-like forbearance which can make one feel very humble.

Outside agencies to which the nurse might want to refer people also have an organisational set-up, details of which ought to be known. It is all very well, for instance, suggesting Marriage Guidance or the local church as possible sources of help, but before doing so one ought to know how well equipped they are to give assistance at that particular time. A woman of my acquaintance once told me of how, when her marriage appeared to be foundering, she eventually nerved herself to contact Marriage Guidance only to discover that in her area – a large industrial conurbation – the service did not operate in the month of August. Similarly a young mother whose baby had been a victim of the 'cot death' syndrome, in her grief felt the urge to go and sit in a church. In the small town where she lived the Methodist, Congregationalist and Anglican buildings were each securely locked.

There is no intention to apportion blame in either of these incidents. Marriage Guidance workers need a holiday as much as anyone else, and if more people offered their services to voluntary movements such problems would not arise. Also, this is an age when lack of parental control, boredom, etc. have made vandalism regrettably commonplace, so many churches have felt the need to lock their premises. If one is neither a regular attender nor gives financial or other support then it is questionable whether one has any right to condemn the practice of keeping church premises locked.

It is probably important for the occupational health nurse to recognise that she does not have the sole prerogative when it comes to counselling, nor, if she is wise, will she attempt exclusiveness in this sphere any more than she would in the realm of safety, where there is a clearly defined chain of interest and responsibility shared with safety, fire and training officers, shop stewards, occupational hygienists, safety representatives and line managers. The nurse may not even have counselling as part of her official job description, and indeed in a large organisation there may be a professional counsellor in post. Nevertheless, it frequently happens that whatever formal structure is devised in an organisation, an informal one grows up alongside it, knowledge of which greatly facilitates achieving one's ends. The nature of the problem may well dictate whose help is sought, and although the nurse will obviously want to give her support in line with official provision, each problem should be looked at as a separate entity.

It has already been implied that prompt resolution is more likely to be the exception than the rule; nevertheless there is perhaps a tendency to see the client in counselling as presenting what might be called an 'acute' condition i.e. suddenly arising and, hopefully, quickly dealt with by competent surgery. There are, however, long-term problems, chronic situations which, by the very complexity of their nature, tend to recur in slightly different forms. For instance, the worker with a chronic disability will sometimes find the attitude of his fellow workers difficult. Many people are frightened of illness and the daily sight of someone with chronic ill health, even reasonably controlled, is more than they can cope with. Consequently they build a shell of indifference, perhaps to deal with their own vulnerability, and avoid contact with the disabled person who begins to see himself as being treated as an outcast. Such a situation is, hopefully, extreme and there will always be mature people who do not react in this way but there is enough reality in the example to give the occupational health nurse cause for thought when the chronically sick worker appears to be unhappy. As those who work in the psychiatric field are wont to say, 'The member of a "family" who presents for treatment is not necessarily the one who is most ill.' Once again, the overall view is one which only the nurse who knows both her work place and work force will fully be able to appreciate. Formal counselling may take place in the Occupational Health Unit but an equal amount can happen informally on routine visits to the shop floor.

The need for redundancy counselling is, unfortunately, increasingly a feature of present day industrial life. It may well be that the problem is on so large a scale that the organisation concerned sets up a special scheme to deal with it. Such a scheme would have three main functions: to provide effective means of communication of information so that everyone affected knows what is happening at any particular stage; to implement the normal personnel function whereby information is gathered about employees so that the maximum assistance could be given, bearing in mind the needs of the organisation and the giving of constructive help towards future employment by helping the employee to recognise his own potential.

It may well be that the nurse has no formal place in such arrangements but it is most likely that she would be involved informally. The experts may well be experts but they are likely to be strangers; the nurse, on the other hand, is the comfortable, familiar individual who over the years has provided solace and strength on a number of occasions. The Occupational Health Unit may well be the place where the information that has been received is re-examined and mulled over, with the nurse acting as sounding board.

The extent to which the effectiveness of an occupational health nurse depends on the information she possesses deserves closer attention. No one can be an expert in all fields, but she can and ought to know who can give the assistance for which she is unqualified by either training or experience. Sources of counselling help would include statutory bodies such as Social Services Departments and Occupational Guidance Units. The former certainly have a counselling function although they tend to be so busy with routine case loads that it receives less time allocation than it should. Occupational Guidance Units, although increasing in number, are not yet widespread, and so their usefulness is limited; where they do operate adults can be assisted to make decisions concerning their careers. Secondly, there are the voluntary bodies, of which in this respect the National Marriage Guidance Council and its Catholic counterpart are the best known. The Samaritans are an obvious related organisation, as are Legal Advice Centres and Pregnancy Advisory services. Another, perhaps under-utilised, resource is the local church. The clergy traditionally have a counselling function, even if the laity are less ready to make use of it than formerly. All the same, it is a potential resource worth investigating. On a personal note I know of at least one minister who has quite an elaborate counselling service operating from his Church centre. Clients are seen without appointment at certain times, by arrangement at others, and discuss problems which range over a very wide spectrum of difficulties covering social as well as spiritual matters. So successful has the service become that referrals from both the Social Services and local general practitioners have become common place. In this instance it is obvious that knowing the workers and the work place includes being aware of the resources in its geographical catchment area too!

By its very nature of confidentiality the counselling role presents certain problems of which the principal one is conflict of loyalties. When legal implications intrude, then the position becomes even more difficult; for instance, the worker who reveals his incapacity for safe working. It is as well for the nurse to have thought through her reaction to such a situation before being faced with it in practice. It may be that sensing the possibility of such a disclosure the nurse might feel compelled to explain to the worker that safety, not only of the man himself but also of his colleagues, would have to take priority of place, before allowing herself to be the recipient of information that would pose such a dilemma. At which point it would seem appropriate to consider some of the inherent problems of the counselling role and what can be done to alleviate them.

It is often maintained that the suicide rate for counsellors and psychiatrists is much higher than the norm.[7] One possible cause of this could be that so many of the problems encountered are incapable of solution and thus the sense of satisfaction, which is one of the main rewards for workers in the caring professions, is absent. It is thus very important that while the counsellor has empathy with her clients she must not identify so closely as to become overwhelmed by them. Not only is this bad for the counsellor's own state of health but it considerably reduces her ability to give help where it is needed. The aim should be a balance between too much identification on the one hand and a remote superiority on the other. Maintaining this balance over many years is no easy problem. One solution, which the clergyman mentioned above practises, is to have one or two people to whom one can go in complete confidence to talk through one's difficulties. The negative energies of the problems are thus to some extent dissipated instead of finding a repository in the counsellor's mind.

The varying needs of different workers have already been identified. It might be appropriate to enlarge on the associated problems which the diverse groups present. The young worker, who has recently left school, will be subject to a variety of new situations, not the least of which may be the change to long hours of perhaps heavy or tedious physical effort, so different from what he has known at school. Some, with more money available to them than ever before, may well go through a rather wild phase before settling down. Young girls, attracted by a mass-media-fostered glamorous view of marriage, often have a very limited view of their future. For both sexes the nurse is frequently the nearest approach to a parent/teacher/confidante that they are likely to encounter.

The worker in his/her twenties and thirties may be beset by money problems resulting from the demands of marriage, mortgages and children. Consequently, as much extra work as possible is taken on to supplement the budget, often at the cost of health and safety. The nurse is quite likely to have experienced or been caught up in a similar situation herself, and thus is able to both understand and keep a watching brief on what is happening. On the other hand, the problems of the middle years of life are often ones of adjustment, accepting where necessary the direction in which life has taken one, and coping with the characteristic physical and mental effects of life at forty plus. In addition, women workers often have two jobs; that of the organisations which employs them, and secondly the demands of their home and family, whether this be as the mother of growing children or as a single woman with an elderly parent.

The older worker, nearing retirement, has a very different kind of problem. He or she needs advice on a variety of matters. If the firm is a large or forward-looking one, then it may well make good provision for those in their sixties, such as special pre-retirement courses, with emphasis on financial advice, health, fitness, leisure, diet, legal matters etc. or schemes which allow retirement to be a gradual process by arranging for an increasingly shorter working week to be worked. Here again, the nurse, whether actively engaged or not, should be aware of what is being offered. Even with the best of schemes the elderly worker may have doubts and worries which can fairly readily be resolved after a chat with the nurse.

There are certain practical points about the actual counselling procedure which are worthy of note. Although much will take place informally, there will be many occasions when a formal counselling situation is more appropriate. When this is the case the following practical suggestions, which are more fully dealt with by Gaynor Nurse in her text book on the subject, are worthy of consideration.

(a) The physical framework of the meeting can be made as helpful as possible. The nurse ought to have an office separate from the surgery for reasons of privacy and confidentiality. As far as possible it ought to have an atmosphere which is pleasant and relaxed. Everyone cannot be skilled with flowers and plants, but for those of us without green fingers, pictures can be a good substitute — horrific safety posters have their place but not in the nurse's office. Desk and chairs should be arranged as informally as possible; indeed, the desk is better out of the way altogether. Most people who are skilled in counselling have a ready supply of tissues and facilities on hand to make tea or coffee. The overall impression should thus be one of welcome and relaxation.

(b) Some people have great difficulty in expressing themselves, particularly when something is troubling them. Consequently, although an opening comment about the weather is a way of breaking the ice, care must be taken that the meeting does not remain fixed at this level. Indeed, some clients may deliberately try to avoid progressing beyond this stage, their courage having failed them at the last moment. It is up to the nurse to recognise what is happening and help the client by asking an open ended question such as, 'What can I do to help you?' Once the client has begun to talk then silence on the nurse's part should be the order of the day, interrupting only where further encouragement is necessary, by such devices as repeating the last comment that the client expressed.

Client: 'No matter how much I do the manager never seems satisfied.'

Nurse: 'You feel the manager does not realise how hard you are working.'

Client: 'Yes, for example. . .' and thus the client is able to continue. Winding up a session can be equally difficult but the important factor is for the ending to have a positive air. If a further meeting would be helpful it should be arranged, if not then the client should feel that he has progressed in resolving his difficulty. If a further meeting is arranged and subsequently the client does not appear, this should be investigated; non-appearance can be a mechanism to avoid further action on an unpleasant matter.

From what has been said in this chapter it will be clear that the nurse who seeks to counsel needs a personal maturity which does not necessarily have anything to do with age, although the ability to cope with the experiences that life sends may well be a good foundation. It is a maturity arising from a sense of humility rather than one of superiority. Her task is not to get people to 'pull themselves together' but rather to recognise how much courage in the face of terrible adversity exists in the world and how this can best be encouraged. Thus, although it is necessary for a counsellor to understand why people behave as they do, it is also necessary for her to be aware of her own faults and limiations.

There is great satisfaction to be gained from helping people, but the important factor is the help one gives to others rather than the self esteem one inwardly fosters. On the other hand, when a problem appears incapable of resolution, the counsellor may feel that she has failed, but this may not be the case. What does matter is that as a counsellor one must be able to accept the occasions when, not only does this happen but, in addition, the failure is commented on by others. A sense of humour and the ability to laugh at oneself are probably among the most important qualities a counsellor might possess, together with a genuine concern for the good of others and patience to await results. People who need help often have a very poor opinion of themselves, certainly subconsciously. The effects of perhaps a lifetime of knocks and disappointments cannot be put right with ten minutes of bracing chat and a cup of coffee. But given time, encouragement and love, the most unlikely plants will blossom.

Notes

1. British Institute of Management, North Staffordshire Branch, 'The Management of Stress Workshop no.4, Preventing the Problems' (unpublished papers, 1978).
2. See Chapter 1.
3. Standing Conference for the Advancement of Counselling, Steering Committee Initial Report (London, 1969).
4. A.H. Maslow, *Motivation and Personality* (Harper & Row, New York, 1954), Chapter 5.
5. F. Herzberg, B. Mauser and B.B. Snyderman, *The Motivation to Work*, 2nd edn. (John Wiley, New York, 1959).
6. Alvin Toffler, *Future Shock* (Pan Books, London, 1971).
7. G. Sworder, 'Problems for the Counsellor in his Task' in A.G. Watts (ed.), *Counselling at Work* (SCAC Bedford Square Press, London, 1977), pp.79-84.

Further Reading

Gaynor Nurse, *Counselling and the Nurse* (HM & M Publishers, Aylesbury, 1975)
A.G. Watts (ed.), *Counselling at Work* (SCAC Bedford Square Press, London, 1977)

8 REHABILITATION

Joyce Bartle

Any reference to the World Health Organisation's definition of health as 'a maintained state of physical, mental and social well-being, and not merely the absence of disease or infirmity', will invariably be followed by an acknowledgement that whilst being the ultimate aspiration, this state will remain elusive to many people and a mythical goal for society as a whole.

The present day emphasis on preventive health care within the population should reduce deviations from the optimal standard of health. Growing awareness of the essential need for individual responsibility for health, and the supporting educative, monitoring and supervisory services within the community have been accompanied by very important and significant advancements in the protection and maintenance of health and safety within the work environment, with vital employer/employee participation and co-operation. With full implementation of recent legislation and, with individual acknowledgement of responsibility for oneself and others, further provision for the protection and maintenance of health within the total environment will be made.

A positive approach towards preventive health care is now the driving force in many branches of nursing and the true *raison d'être* of occupational health nursing. The occupational health nurse is developing her awareness of the objectives of this specialised branch of preventive health nursing: she can see the optimal level of health to be aimed for and maintained. She is, therefore, able to recognise deviations that occur with their varying degrees of physical and psychological trauma on the individual and with their inevitable repercussions on others in the home, the work environment and the organisation. The need to restore the employee to his previous condition as far as possible, and without delay, can be clearly seen.

The necessity for rehabilitative provision in open competitive industry is obvious. In contrast to some of the less tangible, purely preventive health functions, it appears more urgent and beneficial to the employee suffering from some degree of sickness or injury, and to the employer having to cope with the disruption and cost of absenteeism. Much day-to-day rehabilitation is concerned with needs on a small but very significant scale. Whenever a health problem arises at work for an employee, the occupational health practitioner aims to rehabilitate, or 'restore', to normal health and activity.

The nurse's earlier traditional role and her vocational objective were likewise to 'restore' — to rehabilitate — often within the limits of the hospital ward, or perhaps within the community. This was an end in itself; after treatment the patient was considered adequately restored to meet normal everyday demands, and capable of becoming as independent as possible. But little thought was given to his occupation. The occupational health nurse now sees the complete picture of demands within the total environment, of which the diverse and often adverse factors within occupations are amongst the most significant.

The need to relieve discomfort, prevent further impairment, avoid disability and promote rapid, full recovery is equally as important to the employee as it is to the patient, but the function now has an additional purpose; a direct contribution is made to the essential efficiency of the work force and the economic operation of the organisation. It is acknowledged that the benefit/cost ratio of an Occupational Health Service is not easy to evaluate, and the end results certainly must be influenced greatly by the expertise and enthusiasm of the practitioners within the Occupational Health Service — but an organisation financing such a service would no doubt hope for some economic return. The occupational health nurse truly recognises the full scope and value of her place in industry through the necessity for a positive attitude towards the economy and success of the enterprise, with an appreciation of its policies, and the aims and objectives of local managers. With this insight, a rational mind and an acceptance that some limiting factors are bound to exist, opinions can then be expressed, suggestions put forward and every possibility and opportunity pursued and improved upon, towards objective and successful rehabilitation. The benefit to the employee, the employer and the contribution to the economic welfare of the country are both significant and obvious.

Prior to the economic recession in the late sixties the placing of employees into alternative or modified work following injury or, more often, long-term chronic sickness absence, was more common than considered, objective rehabilitation, retraining and resettlement. This would give rise to the creation of supernumerary, 'light work' jobs to accommodate the 'disabled' worker.

Working conditions and living standards of earlier years had no doubt contributed to this lower level of health in some employees. Employees had usually been engaged without initial health screening, and even more significantly, were at times ill-suited to the type of work which they undertook. The health problems of these employees were possibly, during this period, not noted at the time of engagement, and in some cases were exacerbated by the demands and conditions of certain jobs. Employees were therefore frequently working in an environment unsuited to their optimum health. Buildings with several floor levels, steep stairways and often without lifts, with extremes of temperature and industrial dust problems, were examples of this. These alien factors, together with an absence of present-day standards of environmental control and little or no continuum of health supervision, made successful rehabilitation difficult or impossible. Often workers could not cope with the jobs for which they had been employed. In industries where responsibility was accepted, good will existed, and the economic burden could be carried, many light work jobs, such as cleaning and assisting as craftsmen's mates, were created. The earlier 'industrial' nurses faced the situation of workers with health problems in unsuitable occupations. Thus the position of First Aid Attendant was considered suitable light work, despite an absence of training: gatekeepers with chronic health problems were appointed in spite of possible demanding security measures, or patrols which may have had to be carried out in severe weather conditions. Placings were therefore often unsuitable, or uneconomic, when the job was specially created. If retirements had to be made on medical grounds it frequently meant the end of a working career as health was too poor for formal retraining.

Without advisory support, management were at a loss for a satisfactory solution and had no easy task in retaining these 'disabled' employees. The early industrial medical advisers and nurses could make recommendations and give support as far as they were able, but persons specially trained in occupational health and its role in rehabilitation were few. This problem must have been universal. Industrial nurses of that time could see the difficulties experienced by management and the anxiety and despair of the worker struggling with ill-health.

Ironically, it has always seemed that these employees were rarely registered under the Disabled Persons (Employment) Act of 1944, this being seen more as a threat to job security than as helpful protective legislation. They preferred not to identify formally their disability and often chose to accept the severity and permanency of their conditions; no doubt lack of support and fear of financial implications contributed to this. Many industries have failed to maintain the 3 per cent quota of Registered Disabled. However, management could claim that they had a full quota of their own 'disabled' on the payroll by virtue of people going through inevitable periods of ill-health and that these 'disabilities' were considerably more significant than the Registered person whose disability was virtually resolved or was irrelevant to the full, normal job he was doing. The reluctance of these unfit employees to register could be understood; there was little further they could gain by doing so. There was meagre opportunity open to them outside of their own industry and their current employment possibly had the reassuring factor of a sick pay scheme. The two occupations of car park attendant and passenger lift attendant, designated by the Secretary of State for Employment, provided few jobs and required no real skills. Indeed this problem continues to exist today.

Towards the end of the sixties the economic recession with its essential stringencies made it necessary for industry to review its policies, staffing levels, work systems and work force efficiency. In general this caused a need for 'light work' policies to be reviewed. Improved financial provision has been introduced for voluntary redundancy in many instances. State financed unemployment benefit has also increased. This encouraged some of those employees with chronic ill-health to take the opportunity of early retirement. But present-day statistics of man-hours lost from industry through sickness or injury is evidence enough to show the continuing tremendous challenge to health care services.

The World Health Organisation in 1958 summarised the function of medical rehabilitation as having 'The fundamental objective, not only of restoring the disabled person to his previous condition but also of developing to the maximum extent his physical and mental functions'. It is evident that this objective is possible only through a continuum of enthusiastic teamwork. The contribution to be made by today's occupational health nurses in this process is essential to the ultimate success of rehabilitation during the period when communications and co-ordination are particularly liable to break down.

Differing policies resulting from the type of process, the size, economy and philosophy of the employing organisation, cause vastly varying facilities and opportunity for satisfactory rehabilitation. However, regardless of excellent provision, the ultimate result depends on the need being recognised and then being pursued with effort and interest. Industries within which no provision is made must be at a disadvantage in effectively resolving their health problems. Situations no doubt continue to exist where workers with a fair degree of disability struggle to cope with an unsuitable job, lacking the important assessment and supervision, or have prolonged sickness absence without objective guidance, terminating in loss of work potential and lack of suitable resettlement. Additionally, within the smaller firms, long-term absences must have considerable effect, creating a relatively large gap in the work force, with added stress on other workers and a greater impact on the economy of the firm.

Much satisfactory routine rehabilitation must, however, be carried out in open industry, when the occupational health nurse is a key member in the rehabilitation team, often the initiator, investigator, interpreter, innovator and the essential communicator.

All aspects of occupational health practice are integral to the process of rehabilitation. They link the function of health education with its role in advising on reaching full health potential to essential individual participation; health supervision with the need to be alert to remissions; counselling, with the need to give the opportunity for discussion and encouragement to the worker in retaining confidence, self-esteem and self-motivation; environmental control with the nurse's knowledge of work hazards and stresses to ensure that the vulnerable are not put further at risk; therapeutic treatment, and the need for accurate recording of all relevant details of the employee's sickness or injury (including those of a strictly confidential nature) to provide an essential history of the development of the condition; details needed to meet statutory requirements, and statistics necessary for accident and ill-health prevention, epidemiology and research. The functions of communication and co-operation are vital to the rehabilitative process. A valuable and comprehensive exercise of industrial and community interrelations can occur, providing an ideal opportunity for the projection of a less recognised area of nursing, not yet fully acknowledged by management in industry and still less by those working in health care outside of industry.

In addition to the day-to-day rehabilitation of employees with minor sickness or injury, carried out totally within the work environment, there is great need for continuous monitoring of a more serious medical condition or injury, which might involve long-term absence from work. This may have resulted in some level of impairment of bodily function. The impairment may be fairly transient, recovery taking place over a period of time, or the condition can remain permanent, in some instances to a fairly constant degree, in others with periodic acute exacerbation, perhaps resulting in some degree of regression. There are also conditions which will almost certainly progress, such as multiple sclerosis. If the impairment prevents the employee from carrying out his full normal job, the impairment has caused a degree of disability.

The legal definition of a disabled person, contained in the Disabled Persons (Employment) Act of 1944, would apply only to a minority of those employees who benefit from the rehabilitative function of the Occupational Health Service in open industry. The definition describes such a person as 'A person who on account of injury, disease or congenital deformity is substantially handicapped in obtaining or keeping employment, or in undertaking work on his own account, of a kind which apart from that injury, disease or deformity, would be suited to his age, experience and qualifications.'

The primary aim is to rehabilitate the employee back into his own normal full job 'suited to his age, experience and qualifications'. A minority will need retraining and resettlement, and this important aspect is referred to later in this chapter.

Occupational health nurses are likely to accept that rehabilitation starts, ideally, at the onset of illness or injury. Observations made during a study day at Harefield Heart and Chest Hospital, in Hertfordshire (25 May 1978), universally recognised for its quality of care and excellence of success in heart and chest surgery, demonstrate that rehabilitation essentially starts before surgery is undertaken. The patient's health is brought to its optimal level before the operation, and this factor controls the day on which it is considered that surgery should be undertaken. This concept could be applied within industry, by for example, advising the overweight employee or the heavy smoker before a planned hospital admission.

In emergency situations essential First Aid measures can provide the first constructive step towards rehabilitation until more experienced help is forthcoming. The vital insight needed into the immediate care of a worker who could have suffered a heart attack, the caution required for possible spinal injury or the urgency essential to the treatment of burns, are illustrations of this. In less serious day-to-day occurrences, efficient occupational First Aid and nursing care can be seen to have the beneficial effect of assisting rapid rehabilitation with minimal loss of working time. Good initial treatment will prevent complications which can readily occur following injury, such as infection, mallet finger, and frozen shoulder. Improper treatment for an undiagnosed fracture or tendon injury can greatly delay rehabilitation and result in permanent impairment, with possible disability.

It is with the more serious health problems, and those which are liable to cause considerable inconvenience and disruption to the employee and employer, that the function of rehabilitation needs to be approached and pursued with very real enthusiasm, and the obvious needs met. It may be necessary for the employee to be away from work for a considerable time, having to cope with physical and psychological trauma. Individual attitudes and reactions can be seen to vary greatly and the approach towards recovery will be much influenced by the support of his family and his employer.

The nurse's basic training helps her to make some level of preliminary assessment of the severity of the condition, anticipated recovery or long-term or permanent impairment. However, it is sometimes difficult to assess when serious injury or sickness strikes, such as in coronary thrombosis, what the outcome might be. Whilst excessive over-reassurance should not be given, a balanced opinion that a fair recovery and return to work is anticipated is often what the employee needs to hear, to promote essential self-motivation and positive participation in rehabilitation. Frustration, depression and despair are frequently sad accompaniments of these long-term conditions. If some insight and the compassion of nursing care accompanied by objectivity are shown by the occupational health nurse at an early stage, it can be seen that immense support is gained. The personal crisis, unique to the worker, is shared to some measure, and the team work essential to rehabilitation has been initiated.

A small minority of employees could need special medical attention, due to the nature of their illness or injury. Limb amputation and neurological, orthopaedic, cerebro-vascular and psychiatric conditions may benefit from the more specialised rehabilitation available in hospital departments or medical rehabilitation centres, where residential accommodation is often provided. Within these establishments the aim will be to assist the patient to recover fitness, with the additional services of artificial limb and appliance centres, where necessary. The ideal situation would be to have all provision for industrial rehabilitation at the same location, as at Garston Manor, near Watford, Hertfordshire, but these integral facilities are rare.

The illness or injury of the majority of workers, however, permits their medical rehabilitation to take place within the home, thus providing the opportunity for integration with industrial rehabilitation, through occupational health services.

During absence, contact with the work environment can have a strong beneficial influence on the employee, providing continued identification with the work place and opportunity for the supervision of objective, continuing rehabilitation. The contact is especially valuable during depressing long-term illness, when confidence and perseverance, tempered with patience, needs to be encouraged.

Organisations and, indeed, occupational health services, differ in the importance they attach to this aspect of rehabilitative care. Personnel departments, through their Welfare Officers, carry out this responsibility in some instances but the occupational health nurse has the advantage of a background training which enables her to assess the changing medical condition, and to advise on factors influencing satisfactory improvement, leading to re-integration within the work environment. Without this contact a gap in the communications which are essential to positive rehabilitative teamwork is very liable to occur.

The employee should be able to see the nurse in her strictly impartial role, and not as a representative acting on behalf of management emphasising his absence from the work team, and questioning whether his absence is being unnecessarily prolonged. When a justified 'final' medical certificate and return to work is expedited this could be seen as a beneficial development. However, it is important that the nurse's role is not misinterpreted, particularly by those incapable of returning, whilst at the same time a positive approach is essential to minimise unjustified absence, with a lapse in the continuity of rehabilitation.

The family as a whole can at times draw a great deal of support from this communication. Much anxiety can be prevented by allowing discussion of a medical or social problem. Perhaps a close relative, often the wife of an employee, seeks an opportunity for a quiet, confidential word with the occupational health nurse; this support can be very rewarding at a time when many anxieties and uncertainties can exist. If the family unit is already insecure and relationships are unstable, the additional pressures caused by the incapacity result in a stressful atmosphere, with possibly a loss of self-esteem in the worker. If financial or domestic assistance needs to be considered, information could be required on its availability, and the method of obtaining this help, through the Social Services and voluntary organisations, or the Department of Health and Social Security. Welfare services are usually provided within the employing organisation and by close liaison, the nurse can ensure that financial and other personal matters are dealt with – often by the Welfare Officer giving this service in the employee's home as a further member of the rehabilitation team.

The passing of medical information from other health workers, to the occupational health nurse will certainly be limited, and particularly so by telephone conversation, if professional ethics are observed. This restriction might have to be accepted, even though very real concern is felt for an employee in the early days of a serious illness or injury. A hospital or home visit allows objective observation and significant information is frequently volunteered by the employee or relatives. A formal request for medical opinion is often indicated, but usually follows at a later stage, with the employee's written permission, when a more accurate judgement can be made and can be directly related to health and work potential and the assignment to a suitable job.

Informal health education can be indicated during home visits, supporting or complementing that of the general practitioner, or community care services. This can include, for example, advice on diet and weight control, exercise and relaxation. At times, the need for rest and peace of mind is not appreciated by the family, such as when a cardiac condition exists, or there is over-anxiety. The nurse can tactfully attempt to give understanding of the essential needs.

Often the worker has no other regular contact for supervision and assessment. Not infrequently, medical certificates are issued to extend over a three-month period of absence and the patient is left to his own initiative and self-motivation. Early ambulation and discharge from hospital, which is now the rule, could be considered to be on the credit side of satisfactory rehabilitation, but individual responsibility has to be accepted when a good degree of positive restoration must continue, and the occupational health nurse may need to encourage continued self-participation. Occasionally the therapeutic services necessary to successful rehabilitation, such as physiotherapy, occupational and speech therapy, have not been made available and these services must be initiated through the proper channels.

Visits from work colleagues, or perhaps a visit to the work site if the health condition allows, can assist in keeping the employee in touch with 'shop floor' events and a familiar atmosphere, thereby giving psychological preparation for his return.

The health picture will be built up as time passes, and future potential will become more apparent. If the worker can be told that his job is secure, or that modified or alternative work is available — without raising false hopes, and with management confirmation — much undesirable anxiety will be allayed. The employee could well have children and other dependants to support and a mortgage to finance. To be able to work is very significant to him both socially and morally.

Return to work needs to be considered and seen to materialise at the earliest opportunity if full rehabilitation is not to be delayed. That 'work is Nature's best physician' (Galen) is well demonstrated in industrial rehabilitation. It is also recognised that early settlement of compensation claims could well prevent unnecessarily long absences, with their very significant effect on the physical and psychological restoration of the worker and cost to the employer.

A full assessment of the health condition and work ability will be necessary, prior to the employee's return to work. The insight gained by the nurse throughout the absence will enable her valuable opinion to be added to that of the medical advisers.

Where occupational health nurses work without occupational medical support, this contribution is even more crucial because of the need for managers to receive advice, in order to enable them to determine a suitable job assignment. All of the medical information which has been obtained, with the employee's written consent, from his own doctor and possibly the consultant, will combine with that of the occupational health team to provide the relevant factors in relation to the worker's health and his job. In turn, the general practitioner will require to be made aware of the nature of the work available and the provision for health supervision within the work environment. More medical practitioners outside of industry are no doubt asking 'What is your occupation?', but are they aware of the true nature of these occupations and the physical and psychological demands to be matched against the health of the patient?

Sir Ronald Tunbridge, in his Report on Rehabilitation,[1] stated that 'the degree to which rehabilitation is possible and successful will depend not merely on the individual's age and general mental and physical health, but also on the kind of work and mode of life he is expected to pursue'.

The 'kind of work' now pursued, with its effect on the mode of life of the worker, becomes the vital influence on 'possible and successful rehabilitation', All health factors have to be taken into account, being essential to the type of work the employee can undertake. These might include: the degree of cardiac compensation (following coronary thrombosis) or the presence of continuing symptoms when considering manual or mentally stressful work; limited movement or power as a result of neurological, muscular or skeletal conditions, when climbing or the manipulation of machinery is an integral part of the job; and the degree of recovery following hernia repair when heavy lifting is required.

Only when the occupational health nurse has knowledge of the demands of the various jobs can she fully contribute to this aspect of rehabilitation or resettlement. Full discussion with the employee is essential in order that all implications are understood. Thus, for example, a change of job may be considered, perhaps at a lower grade, or with less status or changed rate of pay, and if certain concessions are to be made for a limited period only, say until reassessment, this must be clarified.

Managers require medical recommendations which state what the employee is capable of doing, in addition to any necessary reservations. A positive report eases the task of useful placement, to the satisfaction of employee and employer. Supervisors cannot feel confident with ambiguous recommendations, feeling unable to use the worker to his full capacity, or, through lack of clarity, being liable to place unsuitable demands on him. Managers need to have ideas and suggestions put to them, and they in turn should inform the occupational health staff of job availabilities.

To be enabled to play their important part in rehabilitation, the employer and the work department supervisors need to know when the worker will be returning, in order to plan, if necessary, any special or modified work environment. Most occupational health nurses will have seen the unsatisfactory situation when the employee arrives back on to the work site without warning and when no provision for the required rehabilitation has been co-ordinated. A final certificate, with a request for light work from the general practitioner, places both supervisor and worker at a disadvantage.

A helpful atmosphere in the work environment can make a very significant contribution to successful re-integration. Work colleagues can be anxious and over-protective and, more rarely, resentful, if special concessions have been made to someone receiving equal financial reward. These tendencies have to be rationalised as far as possible. Work problems, as far as confidentiality allows, can be discretely sorted out, and an awareness given of the unobtrusive support that could be helpful and acceptable. Should a problem be liable to arise, to cause anxiety, the method of obtaining help should be clarified.

Rehabilitation of employees within industrial incentive schemes can present a further challenge. Within the schemes there are often wider job demands, with more flexibility required in the application of skills, causing new pressures on those with health problems. The best possible health potential has to be reached, with much emphasis on its maintenance, through health education and self-help and motivation of the worker, and through supervision by the nurse. Nevertheless an important factor is the acceptance of a less able colleague into a work group, The nurse can often 'feel the way' and help in this integration, without breaking confidences and loyalties, or undermining the worker's self-esteem.

To assist the continuum of rehabilitation and a smooth transition from the home environment to the more demanding work atmosphere, special considerations could be necessary. Initially, day work instead of changing shift rotas, or a shorter working day, could perhaps be considered by management. The employee will often find that even limited duties will make far more physical demands on him than is anticipated. Transport might be difficult, perhaps with driving a car, starting a motor cycle or coping with severe weather conditions, following cardiac conditions. The nurse can perhaps initiate alternative transport before the return to work, possibly through the co-operation of another employee.

A basic understanding of ergonomics is important to the nurse, to enable her to assess whether the job suits the changed or reduced functions of the worker. For example, machines can perhaps be modified, or sitting facilities provided. The work can be placed at a different level, for instance, to reduce cervical spine stresses. Handrails could be necessary to protect those with multiple sclerosis, and their work arranged at the ground floor level, with convenient facilities. A small trolley for transporting heavy equipment could reduce the stress on damaged shoulder joints or assist to reduce strain, when other debilities exist. Industries with special physiotherapy units are comparatively rare, but much useful supervised exercise to suit the worker can be continued within the Occupational Health Department, at periods convenient to the work plan.

Redressings may still be required as may suitable provision for stoma care. Occupational health nurses, being aware of accepted professional guidelines, will recognise the need to follow the agreed procedures for certain types of treatment. This type of support and assistance, usually initiated by the occupational health nurse, does much to reduce the stress of coping with physical and psychological impairment in a demanding environment. 'Tis not enough to help the feeble up, but to support him after.' The nurse now recognises, as did Timon of Athens, the essential need for continued support to bring about full rehabilitation.

The employee needs to know that he has confidential assistance available in the medical department, particularly following such conditions as psychiatric illness, alcoholism, or drug dependence. Provision of contact, and the knowledge that the nurse will have time to listen to him, is very vital. It does, without doubt, assist in preventing further breakdown in difficult times when the employee fears he is not coping and becomes withdrawn.

Continuing unobtrusive supervision from the 'sidelines', with regular medical assessments and encouragement of confidence, self-motivation and full participation are now essential strategies. The aim will be for the employee to resume his full, normal work load as soon as his condition allows. Managers need regular reports in order to employ the worker in the correct capacity and to use his full ability with confidence.

Signs of relapse may occur, or the worker's impairment makes it apparent that he is permanently restricted. Conditions such as multiple sclerosis and rheumatoid arthritis are a particular problem, with the need for gradual 'resettlement' into an adapted work environment.

An alternative suitable job, if available within the firm, and if possible amongst his own colleagues, is often in the best interests of the employee. The nurse is sometimes able to see suitable vacancies arising, and can discuss their suitability with managers, with a view to the resettlement of a disabled worker. She should be aware of the continual shift of the health level and potential work ability in the impaired or disabled worker.

Few organisations have the special provision of enclaves, or sheltered workshop conditions. These environments assist greatly in the employment of the disabled alongside their able-bodied colleagues, but are the exception rather than the rule and are not part of the work environment of the majority of occupational health nurses.

The disabled person, if given an opportunity to carry out a satisfying and suitable job, will usually endeavour to retain his status, albeit at a new level, and will fulfil his work role to his own self-esteem and his employer's satisfaction. Physical and psychological trauma can often be considered to have contributed to added strength of character and determination. When statistics showing time lost from work are studied, it can often show that irresponsible attitudes of able-bodied workers are a greater, but less often appreciated,problem.

If resettlement into a suitable job within the organisation is not possible, retirement on medical grounds could become necessary, or if the worker is considered to be suitably fit and likely to be able to take up full employment at the end of it, rehabilitation through statutory or voluntary services could be indicated. The inability to continue with his normal job is almost certain to be psychologically traumatic to the worker. Similar situations can arise following plant closures, with consequent redundancies. Employees with health problems find it extremely difficult, or impossible, to obtain work of a suitable type. Their anxiety for the future can be understood, with the realisation of loss of status, and fear of taking up a dependent role instead of a supportive one, within their families.

The opinion is sometimes expressed that unnecessary emphasis is placed by society on the importance of 'earning' as the only acceptable role, and that for the disabled outside of competitive industry, job satisfaction and quality of life are more important. This assumes that adequate alternative financial provision is made to ensure a satisfactory standard of living. Most workers who have been participating in normal work previously, however, do not readily accept this concept for themselves. They see themselves as the 'breadwinner' and balance a fair wage against their skills and effort. They usually feel the need to fulfil this role and their side of the bargain if it is within their ability. The importance of full rehabilitation from a psychological aspect can thus be seen. When the disability truly prevents this, the occupational health nurse has a special part to play in its acceptance by the worker.

Knowledge of services from which the worker could benefit is of much importance. A complete change of future outlook and quality of life — summed up by Mr Alfred Morris, Minister for the Disabled, during the second reading of his Chronically Sick and Disabled Persons Bill, as 'adding life to years' — could result from sound guidance and encouragement given at a time when a fresh look has to be taken regarding future employment and independence.

Since the last war four Government Committees in the United Kingdom have spent much time reviewing rehabilitation services and yet a dichotomy of responsibility for rehabilitation remains. The Department of Health and Social Security (1966) deals with medical rehabilitation, that is, for the patient, of any age group whereas the Department of Employment (1968) deals with Industrial Rehabilitation, now through the independent Manpower Services Commission (1974), for the working population.

Occupational health nurses who have studied the latest of the four Reports by the Sub-Committee at the Standing Medical Advisory Committee of the Central Health Services Council, under the Chairmanship of Sir Ronald Tunbridge, in 1972, will be aware of its far-reaching recommendations for a fully comprehensive rehabilitation service. There was also much criticism of the lack of training in the speciality and of the absence of enthusiasm and effort, communication and co-ordination.

In many areas these inadequacies still persist, to frustrate those who are in need and those who are aware of the gaps and deficiencies. Economic restrictions have no doubt contributed to lack of progress and the depressed employment situation has not created a demand for manpower with the full use of the disabled.

In some districts, however, a good deal of initiative and a positive attitude towards medical rehabilitation exists and the Manpower Services Commission has made further provision for industrial rehabilitation. A wide range of information on present day rehabilitation, retraining and resettlement services is available through the Employment Services Agency[2] and up-to-date literature can give a comprehensive picture of the excellent organisations and establishments throughout the country.

If opportunity arises for occupational health nurses to study at these establishments, greater awareness of the facilities available to the workers can be gained. In addition opportunity is provided to project the essential and much underestimated contribution that occupational health teams can make. More involvement with employers at this level, and a more rigid enforcement of the required disabled quota, could no doubt lead to a more objective contribution to full rehabilitation and resettlement in open industry, where a suitable environment exists.

The occupational health team's contact for initiating this type of retraining and resettlement, in co-ordination with the worker's own doctor, is the Disablement Resettlement Officer, of the Employment Services Agency: his service is available to all disabled people and those who employ or intend to employ them. His aims are to encourage employers to take disabled people into jobs they will do well, and with satisfaction, and to ensure that the disabled, or those who are no longer able to undertake their usual occupation because of industrial change, make full use of available opportunities.

If an employee is disabled within the meaning of the Disabled Persons (Employment) Act of 1944, and the disability is likely to last for at least twelve months, and the person wishes to work, with a likely prospect of being able to do so, the nurse can explain to him the advantage provided by registration. The Disablement Resettlement Officer will be able to give details of employers' duties regarding the employing of a percentage of registered disabled workers, and vacancies for designated jobs under the Order of 1946, but, as illustrated earlier, employers tend not to comply with the legislation of a quota system and the designated jobs are limited in availability and skills. However, the training or employment in Remploy's sheltered workshop and in those of some of the local authority and voluntary organisations is usually reserved for persons on the Register. In addition, those registered as severely disabled are eligible for certain special facilities. Disablement Resettlement Officers will also be aware of suitable and congenial job opportunities and this could lead to satisfactory resettlement.

Formal industrial rehabilitation and expert assessment is provided in the 26 United Kingdom Employment Rehabilitation Centres. A Centre Manager, an Employment Medical Adviser who is often assisted by a nurse, remedial gymnasts, an occupational psychologist, a social worker, a Disablement Resettlement Officer and a Chief Occupational Supervisor, form an expert team. A consultant psychiatrist is also available if required. Tax-free maintenance allowances, assistance with fares, lodging allowances and National Insurance contributions are paid to clients during the courses, which last on average about six weeks. At the end of this time the person would be prepared and assessed for suitable re-employment or further training.

If it is felt that the disabled person could benefit, opportunities can be gained from Training Opportunity Schemes provided by the Training Services Agency. Courses are offered in a variety of skilled or semi-skilled occupations. These are held at Skillcentres and other educational centres, or industrial premises and at residential training colleges, for the severely disabled; allowances similar to those of the Employment Rehabilitation Centres are provided.

These services aim to enable the disabled person to contribute once again in suitable, open industry, or sheltered employment. The occupational health nurse could find that these opportunities could benefit a worker unable to be rehabilitated within his normal work environment.

The results of various studies and surveys on the impaired and disabled and their employment give evidence of the scale of disability as a social and economic problem. In 1967 1½ million citizens in the United Kingdom were officially described as disabled or handicapped.[3] These made up 3 per cent of the total population. A later survey carried out in 1968-9 by Amelia Harris[4] and her colleagues at the Social Survey Division of the Office of Population Censuses and Surveys, found that there were just over 3 million impaired people over the age of sixteen living in private households.

The Chronically Sick and Disabled Persons Act (1970), which placed further responsibility on the Social Services Departments, recommended that more local awareness should be developed and further facilities made available. Public expectations were encouraged by legislation, but at the same time local authorities' public expenditure cuts had been made. Between March 1973-4 there was a 25 per cent increase in the number of handicapped on the local authorities' 'general classes'

Register; no doubt this increase was due to local surveys following the 1970 Act.[5]

To the health care practitioners working in Occupational Health Services, the numbers of unemployed disabled of working age would appear particularly significant. A fall in the level of employment, with increased competition for work, drastically affects the disabled. Jn 1976 unemployment rates of Registered Disabled were over 13 per cent and represented 70,000 people. The disabled formed nearly one in fifty of the working population, but at the same time they were also one in sixteen of the total unemployed.[6] These figures demonstrate the vital need for preventive health medicine to produce positive results, with Occupational Health Services making a very significant contribution. Alfred Morris commenting on the philosophy behind the Chronically Sick and Disabled Persons Bill, remarked that 'what most disabled people want more than anything else is to lessen their dependence on other people, to get on with living their own lives as normally as they can in their own homes, amongst their own families, and whenever possible, to have the opportunity of contributing to industry and society as fully as their abilities allow'. Industry can contribute considerably to this philosophy.

Within the Employment Medical Advisory Service of the Health and Safety Commission progress has been made in developing occupational nursing services within Employment Rehabilitation Centres and Skillcentres. Senior Nursing Advisers have as one of their special responsibilities the maintaining of liaison with rehabilitation and retraining establishments and for advising the Senior Employment Medical Adviser concerned with rehabilitation and mental health, on nursing factors. In 1976 a specialist Employment Nursing Adviser post was created for a research assistant in rehabilitation; the nurse works with the Senior Medical Adviser for Rehabilitation and Fitness for Work, who is responsible for the co-ordination of advice on medical aspects of health in relation to occupation, and on rehabilitation, retraining and resettlement, organised by the Manpower Services Commission.

The need for occupational health nurses to have specialised knowledge and expertise is now recognised by the Nursing profession; managers in industry are also beginning to acknowledge the importance of the availability of expert supportive advice on matters of health and the environment. The Royal College of Nursing has increased its commitments to occupational health and the provision of specialised training.

The first two professional University Chairs of Rehabilitation in the United Kingdom established at Southampton and Edinburgh acknowledge the need for development and training and the recent creation of a Faculty of Occupational Health within the Royal College of Physicians should assist further in the understanding and acceptance of the value of occupational health care. The Employment Training Act 1973, through the Manpower Services Commission 1974, has made a wider range of services available under the Employment Services Agency and Training Services Agency.

The urgent necessity for research and actual development in the field of rehabilitation appears to be gaining recognition. That 'reports are not self executive'[7] has been well demonstrated by the lack of full implementation of earlier legislation and the failure to develop recommendations of former Reports. Perhaps, at the present time, the growth of the function of rehabilitation is becoming more of a reality and will be seen to fulfil a desperate need.

At a time of rapid development in medical technology, there continues to be the basic need to give the full quality of life to individuals. When sickness and injury occur, the maximum restoration to health to enable the carrying out of a suitable job is necessary to fulfil this need.

The continuity and success of full rehabilitation are dependent on the integration of medical and industrial rehabilitation, both at statutory level and through co-ordinated effort between Occupational Health Services and Health Care Services outside of industry. It is through the latter partnership, and by increased awareness of society of all available services, that a major part of day-to-day rehabilitation will be successfully achieved.

The teamwork of rehabilitation embraces every facet of occupational health nursing but is a function of singular importance. If this became recognised and practised to its full effect throughout industry, with the occupational health nurse in a key role, the social and economic results on individual workers and their families, other employees, employers and society as a whole would be far-reaching and very considerable.

Notes

1. Sir Ronald Tunbridge, Report of Sub-Committee of Standing Medical Advisory Committee, Central Health Services Council (HMSO, London, 1972).
2. Manpower Services Commission, Employment Services Agency, *Rehabilitation, Retraining and Resettlement* (HMSO, London, 1976).

3. P. Townsend, *The Disabled in Society* (Royal College of Surgeons, 1976).
4. A.I. Harris *et al.*, 'Handicapped and Impaired in Great Britain, Part 1', Office of Population Censuses and Surveys (HMSO, London, 1971).
5. DHSS, *Health and Personal Social Service Statistics for England 1975* (HMSO, London, 1976).
6. P. Townsend, *Poverty and Low Incomes amongst Disabled People;* and A. Walker *Living Standards in Crisis* (The Disability Alliance, London, 1977).
7. Miss F. Nightingale, Marginalia on the draft of the Report of the Sanitary Commission on the Health of the Army (1857).

Further Reading for information on Rehabilitation provisions outside of industry

S. Mattingly (ed.), *Rehabilitation Today* (Update Publications Ltd., London, 1977).

9 CO-OPERATION

June Homewood

The success of any service depends on the ability of its staff to build inter-personal relationships, establish communication channels, co-ordinate and monitor the service and co-operate with others involved with the provision of facilities and personnel. Professional isolation can inhibit the development of Occupational Health Services because occupational health nurses often work alone and lack specialised training. This feeling of isolation may stem too from the fact that there is no national Occupational Health Service and nurses having trained in the National Health Service (NHS) are then practising on their own; also the government responsibility for occupational health rests with the Department of Employment (DE) and not the Department of Health and Social Security (DHSS), and this has resulted in NHS staff having little or no education in understanding the practice of occupational health and may have limited the natural communication which should take place between the two services.

However, staff are only as isolated as they allow themselves to be; there is no need at all to remain in professional isolation as it is now possible in most parts of the United Kingdom to obtain specialised education, and it is always possible to read widely and to keep in touch with one's colleagues and professional organisation. Professional integration is open to all motivated occupational health nurses and is essential in the maintenance of high standards of practice which includes co-operation with all people that are concerned with the promotion of health and safety.

Occupational Health Centres are based in the community albeit the working community and are involved in the provision of primary health care. Colleagues in community health use the term 'primary health care' when referring to the first point of contact between a member of the public and the community based health services, each member of the various health care disciplines having their own specific skills to bring to the Primary Health Care Services.[1] Since occupational health nurses constitute the first point of contact that workers have with a health care discipline they, by definition, deliver primary health care in the same way as do their colleagues in the Primary Health Care Teams. Occupational health nurses are advantaged since to some extent they

148

have a captive audience; they know where and when a worker can be found during the course of a working day and can plan informal 'care' accordingly; whereas health visitors and social workers are reliant on people being available at home and willing to be seen as presenting to the NHS or local authority (LA) to be in need of care.

So it can be seen that occupational health nurses who integrate with other necessary services and achieve maximum co-operation are ideally placed to co-ordinate care for the clients/patients they serve. The speciality of occupational health has been so divorced from most other health and social services that its success revolves around the occupational health nurse's ability to express her aims and objectives to the members of the health care team. When this is achieved a two way co-operation will also be achieved.

Team Concept

Occupational health nurses are employed to deliver occupational health nursing care; to do this well they need to co-operate in various ways:

1. as employees with an employer;
2. with other workers within an Occupational Health Department;
3. with a team of occupational health safety and welfare specialists;
4. with managers of other departments;
5. with outside agencies.

All employees need to understand and respect the terms and conditions of employment that were initially negotiated with the employer; occupational health nurses have the same responsibility to co-operate with the employer as any other employee. Additionally, occupational health nurses as professional people need to maintain the independence, impartiality and confidentiality that is required of them. Successful co-operation at this level depends largely on the nurse's ability to negotiate terms and conditions of employment at her initial interview with the employer. It will also depend on the acceptance by management, union and other health professionals of an agreed occupational health policy. Nurses who are untrained in this speciality or who are applying for their first post in occupational health should seek guidance from their professional organisation before they attend for interviews, for it is at this stage of career development that occupational health nurses need the support of their profession. Occupational health nurses are either based in Occupational Health

Centres or they give a visiting service to companies who provide occupational health facilities. In either case they are part of a team which may include doctors and nurses. A nurse can be manager of that team, a team co-ordinator or a subordinate member of the team. Large organisations have teams which may include a number of doctors, State Registered and Enrolled Nurses, First Aiders, clerks, cleaners and visiting chiropodists, physiotherapists, dentists etc., whilst small organisations may employ just one nurse and a number of auxiliary First Aiders. The team that has evolved will be the one that was developed to forward the agreed occupational health policy of that concern. The nurse like other team members should be loyal to her colleagues, be able to develop good inter-personal relationships and understand the individual strengths and weaknesses of the group of people with whom she works. Like others in the team, she must be committed to the aims and objectives established within the company policy, the success of which will be determined by the degree of co-operation achieved by the team.

The occupational health team is also part of a larger company team which has an interest in health and safety at work and the successful implementation of the Health and Safety at Work etc., Act 1974, which itself relies on the total commitment of all working people for its success. This team has representatives from the personnel, training, security, safety, fire and welfare departments as well as from the trade unions; occupational hygienists, ergonomists, health physicists, occupational psychologists and engineers may also be involved. In order to function alongside these disciplines, occupational health nurses must be able to achieve the same professional standards as their colleagues, and they must have a thorough understanding of the past experience and training of each individual team member, so that as and when necessary they are able to draw on the expertise of their colleagues. It is also essential that the members of the team understand the contribution that the nurse has to offer. Multidisciplinary teams may find it harder to adjust to teamwork than single disciplinary teams since they did not train together and do not always understand their position within the team and therefore find it difficult to achieve high standards of co-operation.

Whether the nurse is the manager of the Occupational Health Department or not, there will be times when it becomes her responsibility to communicate information to departmental managers and gain their co-operation. Therefore, it is essential that she is fully conversant with the names, designations and roles of these managers and that she knows when and where to find them. Normally these facts are available to the nurse when she attends the company induction course. When the nurse has not undergone an induction course, she should make it her business, early in her employment, to meet all the members of the management team as well as the convenors and shop stewards. Once this is done, the correct information can be communicated to the correct people. In addition to this, the nurse will have established her identity, role and function and, in time, will be fully aware of each manager's responsibilities; this will enable management and unions to co-operate with her and ensure that she too receives the day-to-day information that she needs.

Sometimes occupational health nurses will be faced with problems that cannot be resolved either by her or other specialists within the work place; because of this there will always be a need for nurses to work with outside agencies, which mainly fall into one of four definite systems, which will be described later in this chapter. Here it should be emphasised that it is impossible to obtain the necessary help and co-operation from these services unless the occupational health nurse understands their structure, functions and limitations, keeps herself up to date with current social policy and the industrial system and is prepared to introduce herself to the local services.

The occupational health nurse's role in health education has been described in Chapter 6. Of primary importance is the role of the nurse as an educationist, both withing the organisation that employs her and with outside agencies. She continuously needs to make people aware of the concept of occupational health and, when this two way education is established and maintained, co-operation is more likely to be achieved.

Outside Agencies

By using the process of nursing, occupational health nurses are better able to assess when they need to make use of outside agencies, yet they must, of course, be aware of the structure and functions of the agencies that may be essential to complement and supplement the client/patient care that the work place itself is able to offer. It is also essential that management is approached before outside agencies are invited into the work place and that it is the client/patient that accepts the necessity to use an outside agency following either counselling or advice from the nurse.

Under this category of outside agencies, four different systems can be described and there are advantages and disadvantages with each system. (The Future of Voluntary Organisations, 1978, p.22.)[2]

First, there is the informal system of 'social helping'. This is the help and support that family, friends and neighbours give to each other and consists mainly of provision of care of children, sick people, the handicapped and the elderly, as well as advice and psychological support in times of need, e.g. birth, marriage, death and divorce; financial help and gifts to those who are in relative poverty. Occupational health nurses who have ascertained from clients their past history, family history and occupational history should be aware of how much social help clients/patients are expected to offer and can expect to receive in given situations. The evolution of the symmetrical family[3] has meant that not every family can rely on this informal system since the extended family is not now the established norm and in some social classes families are expected to move frequently to achieve promotion prospects at work. Help that is available from the informal system needs to be measured and assessed when planning total patient care, to ensure that the correct outside agency is approached for co-operation and help.

Secondly, there is the commercial system which provides for a whole range of private services e.g. education, pensions and housing for members of society that are able and willing to afford them. Within this category are many information and advisory services that can be available to the occupational health nurse as to her employer and are described fully in the book *Occupational Health. A Guide to Sources of Information* (1974).[4] Another area of this system is for the day-to-day family support of dual career families, with regard to housekeepers, child minders, cleaners and gardeners etc.

Thirdly, there is the statutory service which, in 1975, accounted for 53.5 per cent of all central and local government expenditure and is now so well established that the use of the other systems can be neglected. The advantages of this system are that: there is national coverage, risk is shared in that those in need are supported by the rest of the community, equal treatment for all should be available, standards are maintained, staff are usually selected and qualified and that the services are integrated and controlled in principle. However, there are very real disadvantages; the cost of provision is escalating, demand still exceeds provision of service, statutory services are slow to change, suffer the disadvantages of bureaucracies and can be inflexible, integration has never been achieved and the lay public feel that these services are remote and impersonal.

Fourthly, there exists the voluntary system which complements, supplements and influences the informal, the statutory and the commercial systems. The Wolfenden Report[2] suggests that the voluntary system contributes in three ways: first by identifying need and innovating new services it traditionally extends state services (e.g. The Family Planning Association); secondly, the choice of service is extended and a voluntary service may be acceptable to a client/patient who has rejected statutory services; thirdly the sum total of the , resources available is extended. The advantages of this system are that it is informal, flexible, is available where no statutory service yet exists and it can innovate and change policy very quickly in comparison with the statutory system. The disadvantages are that there is no even distribution of service, performance is variable, many staff are untrained, standards vary and not all needs are met. There is often duplication and overlap between voluntary services and they rely on voluntary financial help and/or state help which varies according to the national economy and can be withdrawn.

The use of outside agencies is sometimes essential and therefore the occupational health nurse must become an expert at choosing the correct system to use and in co-operating with the service that the agency provides and the individual specialists within each agency. Therefore, when needing to co-operate with an outside agency occupational health nurses need to assess not only which system will be of most value to the client/patient, but also which is the quickest, most flexible and most efficient; as well as the most acceptable to the individual concerned.

For the purposes of this book the statutory services that occupational health nurses are most likely to use will be briefly described and the roles of the specialists she will need to co-operate with will be described in more detail. It is impossible to describe and discuss here each of the voluntary services that may be useful to the clients/patients of the occupational health nurse. It is better that nurses learn the current trends in health and social problems and keep up with the continuing changes so that they are well able to discern which clients/patients in the working population are more likely to present with problems. If this is done and adequate up-to-date reference books which describe the voluntary services are to hand, then occupational health nurses should have the basic information they need.

Statutory Services

The statutory services that occupational health nurses need to know of and learn to co-operate with mostly relate to the Department of Employment (DE), the Department of Health and Social Security

(DHSS), the Local Authority (LA) and the Department of Education and Science (DES).

The Department of Employment

The Secretary of State for Employment is responsible to the Government for the Department of Employment which is divided into three main branches.

1. The Health and Safety Commission.
2. Manpower Services Commission.
3. The Conciliation and Arbitration Service.

The Health and Safety Commission. This was established on 1 October 1974 under the Health and Safety at Work etc., Act 1974 (HASAWA) with a full time chairman and between six and nine part-time members consisting of representatives drawn from employers, employees, trade unions and specialists from other organisations including local authorities. Very briefly its duty is to keep the Secretary of State for Employment informed of its work and carry out his directions, ensuring that adequate advice and information on health and safety matters are available, that research and training are undertaken as necessary and that new regulations are prepared when needed. It can arrange for routine investigations and inquiries and obtain any information needed to carry out its functions. It can also approve and issue Codes of Practice containing practical guidance made by itself and prepared by other bodies. It should be remembered that one of the purposes of the HASAWA was to tidy up the many regulations made under the Factories Act 1961 and that it will eventually supersede the Factories Act and the Offices Shops and Railway Premises Act 1963. Regulations, orders, codes of practice and notes for guidance will be made over the next few years and it is part of the occupational health nurse's duty to co-operate and ensure that this legislation is complied with. A good and current example of this is the Safety Representatives and Safety Committees Regulations 1977 (SI 1977 no. 500).[5] HMSO currently publish the 'Regulations, Code of Practice and Notes for Guidance' together in one booklet and this is a useful example of how people at work will be informed and guided in the future. The Health and Safety Executive was established on 1 January 1975 under the HASAWA. It is responsible to the Commission for carrying out its function according to the directions it has received. It has a specific duty to make adequate arrangements for the enforcement of the statutory provision.

From time to time, occupational health nurses will need to seek advice from the Health and Safety Executive and its inspectors, and co-operate with them. Therefore, they should understand the powers which they have, which are set out in Section 146 of the Factories Act 1961.

Occupational health nurses together with the health and safety team should be aware of the advice the Inspectorate has given the employer and of any improvement or prohibition order that has been made. The nurse has a duty to co-operate as an *ex-officio* member of the health and safety team. She may be involved in the inspection of the work places together with the safety representatives, her duties including either keeping or supervising the keeping of statutory records (e.g. accident book, general register, health register which the Inspectorate may wish to see). As part of her day-to-day work, the occupational health nurse should co-operate as necessary with the Inspectorate and ensure that management, unions and employees are fully aware of the powers of the Inspectorate and the advisory function they have

The Employment Medical Advisory Service (EMAS) was originally set up under the Employment Medical Advisory Service Act 1972 and became operational on 1 February 1973. The main provisions of this 1972 Act were replaced in 1974 by HASAWA when EMAS became part of the HSE on 1 January 1975 and the Chief Employment Medical Adviser became Director of the HSE's Medical Services. For organisational purposes the service is directed from London and the country is divided into seven English regions in addition to Scotland and Wales. Each region has a Senior Employment Medical Adviser who works with a team of Employment Medical and Nursing Advisers. The objectives of this service defined in a report on its work for 1973 and 1974 are as follows:

> to identify health hazards related to employment, to advise on the extent of environmental control necessary to minimise health risks related to employment, monitor the effect of action taken to reduce the risk, to advise and inform workers and employers of any risk to health to which they may be exposed, to advise the medical aspects of employment problems especially the employment of disabled people and rehabilitation for employment.

Just as the Inspectorate is involved with environmental monitoring, so this service is involved in medical monitoring through statutory and

voluntary medical and biological monitoring; statutory medicals are
sometimes performed by EMAS and sometimes by occupational health
physicians designated by EMAS. It should be noted that whilst the
employer is bound by statute to allow EMAS to examine an employee
and to provide facilities for this, employees have the right to refuse a
non-statutory medical examination. EMAS are also involved in the
'follow up' of young people (those between school leaving age and 18)
whom the school medical service have identified as in need of
surveillance. The success of the EMAS and Occupational Health Services
depends on mutual respect and continuous co-operation in the
teamwork that is essential for the progress of occupational health.
Occupational health nurses will be involved in co-operating with EMAS
both in the routine part of their work and in the epidemiological surveys
and clinical studies which are undertaken. As the results of relevant
surveys are published for EMAS by HMSO, occupational health nurses
should obtain those which are relevant to their work and their work
place.

The Manpower Services Commission. This gained its responsibility for
employment and vocational training services under the Employment
and Training Act 1973, and functions through two bodies: the Training
Service Agency and the Employment Service Agency. The Training
Service Agency is a governmental retraining system which can be used
when employers find retraining of redundant and other workers either
impractical or impossible. Technological progress and economic
development have made it necessary for many organisations to undergo
the process of rationalisation, to enable them to compete in world
markets. This has resulted in a decline in some occupations such as
unskilled workers and a rise in other occupations, e.g. professional
and scientific occupations.[6] Employed and unemployed workers can
be accepted for retraining, the financial allowances payable being in
excess of both unemployment and supplementary benefits. The training
is provided in Skillcentres, Universities, Polytechnics, Colleges of
Further Education and in employers' establishments. The range and
level of the courses is wide and the scheme is known as the Training
Opportunities Scheme (TOPS). This is the scheme by which nurses who
are not employed as occupational health nurses may be financed to
train in this speciality. Practising occupational health nurses should
make the scheme known to clients who may need to retrain.

The Employment Service Agency is concerned with Job Centres and
Employment Offices, as well as the work of Disablement Resettlement

Offices and Employment Rehabilitation Centres. Job Centres have evolved in recent years presenting a new image for government non-employment services. Eventually it is hoped that the work that is connnected with employment that is now effected in Local Employment Offices will all transfer to Job Centres. At the moment both Job Centres and Employment Offices offer the following facilities:

(a) information on jobs currently available;
(b) advice on job opportunities;
(c) occupational guidance (in the main centres only);
(d) a separate service for professional, executive, managerial, technical and scientific appointments known as Professional and Executive Recruitment (in key centres only).

Simultaneously, extramural departments in higher education offer schemes for redundant executives and women wishing to return to employment.

The Employment Service Agency is also responsible for the services for the disabled and these have been described in Chapter 8. Through a thorough understanding of this government provision, occupational health nurses should be able to reinforce the advice that personnel managers have already given employees when they prepare them for redundancy or unemployment. This kind of co-operation between company specialists enhances the client's likelihood of understanding the services that are available to him or her.

The Conciliation and Arbitration Services. As employees, all nurses should have an understanding of modern employment law. Occupational health nurses, as members of a health, safety and welfare team, need a working knowledge of the law which affects employment and, whilst it is not within the scope of this chapter to describe fully the Conciliation and Arbitration Services, it should be emphasised that it is impossible to co-operate with new members of management and employees unless some aspects of this service are understood, since some problems cannot be evaluated without knowledge of legislation.

The Department of Health and Social Security (DHSS)

The Secretary of State for Social Services has the responsibility of the Department of Health and Social Security (DHSS). Since the National Health Service Act 1946, the government have implemented a comprehensive service which aims at maintaining and promoting the health of the population of England and Wales. This service is concerned with both diagnosis and prevention of disease and there are separate acts for Scotland and Northern Ireland.

In order to liaise effectively with the various services provided, occupational health nurses need to understand their structure and functions as well as current changes in policy with regard to the provision of care. At the moment, a Royal Commission on the NHS is studying all aspects of the service and readers will need to acquaint themselves with the findings of the Commission and to appreciate any changes that may be made following this report.

The NHS has three main divisions which are as far as possible integrated.[7]

1. The Personal Practitioner Services.
2. The Hospital Services.
3. The Community Health Services.

1. The Personal Practitioner Service. This service includes doctors, dentists, opticians and chemists and the responsibility for it lies with the Family Practitioner Committees (FPC) who pay practitioners and investigate complaints made against individual practitioners. Their administrative areas are usually coterminous with the new county councils and metropolitan district councils. It is the FPC that enters into contract with the individual practitioner (who is self-employed and not employed by the NHS) and prepares lists of practitioners. These lists may be useful to occupational health nurses who are setting up a new service or who are themselves newly in post. Occupational health nurses will often need to refer clients/patients to practitioners and need to remind new employees to register with a general practitioner. Therefore a list of local practitioners helps clients/patients choose which practice or practitioner they will approach.

It should be appreciated that many practitioners have no knowledge of the location of Occupational Health Services in their district and even less knowledge of the treatment these services may offer or the qualification and training of the staff in the services. Therefore it is useful if occupational health nurses are able to introduce themselves to local practitioners and outline the service that is offered and the hazards of work that may affect the health of the practitioner's patients: they may describe the facilities that are available in the work place which may either enable patients to continue treatment prescribed by the practitioner at work in working time, or facilitate early return to work following illness or accidents. Of the services offered through the FPC the occupational health nurse is likely to refer to the general practitioners more often than the other practitioners.

General practitioners may practise on their own or they may practise within a group. The group practice may sometimes be based on a Health Centre where a number of general practitioners are based together with other health practitioners. Some organisations invite dentists who are contracted to the Family Practitioner Committee to provide NHS treatment on a sessional basis within the occupational health premises: this is very useful in large industries or in special industries such as the food industry where dental hygiene may affect the product; where this is not so, lists should be available to enable patients to choose their dentist and occupational health nurses should liaise with local dentists especially to ensure that emergency treatment is forthcoming when patients need it. During the transition from work to school, occupational health nurses need to see that young people who have previously used the school dental service appreciate the necessity to use the FPC services; the ageing employee who needs education for the use of dentures should be encouraged to go to the dentist and those patients who are entitled to free or reduced NHS payments for any of these services should be made aware of their rights (these include the young, the pregnant, the retired and those in poverty).

Employees approaching middle age who may need spectacles for the first time should be encouraged to see their general practitioner who would make the initial referral to an optician; following this the nurse should co-operate with the practitioner to ensure that regular visits are made. The occupational health nurse should also have a list of chemists who prepare NHS prescriptions and be aware of their opening times and rotas for emergency services.

2. The Hospital Services. The Regional Health Authorities (RHA) are appointed by the Secretary of State and are responsible for the long term planning of hospital buildings and services in each of the 14 NHS regions: each allocates resources between the Area Health Authorities (AHA) within its boundaries. The regional team of officers includes Medical, Nursing and Works Officers, an Administrator and a Treasurer who work with the area teams of officers in the planning and co-ordinating of services. It should be emphasised that the regional team of officers does not 'manage' the area officers.

There are 90 Area Health Authorities which provide a comprehensive health service at area level and have boundaries which are coterminous

with local government boundaries. The area team consists of a Medical
Officer, a Nursing Officer, Treasurer and Administrator who prepare
plans for presentation to the RMA and also plans with local authority
LA) staff, policies to present to the Joint Consultative Committee (JCC)
which has the responsibility of advising on the planning and operation
of the health services and the social, environmental and educational
services run by the local authority. Executive responsibility is delegated
to the District Management Teams (DMT), whilst the area team of
officers retains the responsibility of monitoring the performance and
co-ordinating the activities in each of the districts within the boundary.
There are 'single district areas' but most areas are divided into up to
five districts.

Whilst it is necessary to know how the hospital service functions for
practical day-to-day purposes, it is essential that occupational health
nurses work closely with the services that are provided at district level.
The White Paper Command 5055 (para. 55) states that 'each district
will form the natural community for the planning and delivery of care'.
Each NHS district serves a population of about 250,000 and either has a
District General Hospital and/or group of hospitals, as well as a number
of health centres. At this level the health service is fully integrated and
local professional staff are fully involved in the planning and delivery
of all health care. The DMT is composed of a District Community
Physician, Nursing Officer, Finance and Administrative Officers as well
as selected representatives from the district medical committee, one
hospital consultant and one general practitioner. Each team member has
equal rights and none may override the other. In order to avoid
domination by any member or members of the team, the whole team
has to come to a consensus of opinion on any matter of decision.
Unresolved disagreements must be referred to the AHA.

The NHS Reorganisation Act 1973 established Community Health
Councils (CHC) in each NHS district. The function of the CHC's is to
represent the consumer and his/her views. The councils have rights
enabling them to function adequately, which include: the right to be
consulted; the power to secure information and visit hospitals and
health centres etc; direct access to the AHA. Their role is to assess the
adequacy of the health services provided for the community, comment
on plans for future development and compare how local provision links
into the national picture. The success of these councils depends on the
ability and enthusiasm of the appointed 18 to 30 members and the
motivation of the lay public and professional people who choose to
attend these public meetings. Occupational health nurses could be

members of these councils; they should attend local meetings to keep abreast with local developments and problems in the NHS.

There is a necessity for occupational health nurses to liaise and co-operate with the hospital service since there will always be a small number of patients within the care of an Occupational Health Service who are currently undergoing hospital treatment either as inpatients or as outpatients. Occupational health nurses may be involved in all stages of hospital care. For example, they may have made the initial referral or co-operate by maintaining treatment, health supervision or health education and they will certainly be involved in any resettlement, retraining or rehabilitation that is to take place on or before return to work. In the course of their work, they may visit Casualty Departments in Eye Hospitals and District General Hospitals, be in contact with Outpatient Departments over appointments or treatment and visit wards.

This constant liaison will keep occupational health nurses up to date in current treatments and procedures and will promote an awareness of occupational health as a speciality among all grades of NHS staff.

3. The Community Health Services. The objectives of reorganisation of the NHS under the 1974 Act were to unite the health services, establish close links with LA services, involve the professions and the public in the running of the service and ensure central control over finance through well defined management structures (DHSS National Health Service 1970). The Community Health Services, together with the Practitioner and Hospital Service already described should at District Level provide an integrated service, through the provision of Group Practices, Clinics, Health Centres and Hospitals but the success of this relies on co-ordinating the work. This in turn relies on a team approach with individual members of that team understanding and respecting other members' contributions. Confusion still exists at this level since general practitioners contracted to the NHS can still, if they wish, practise alone or from a group practice or practise from a health centre, yet at the same time may have nursing staff attached to their practice. Alternatively, the nursing staff may be directly employed by the NHS.

Also, there is now some confusion concerning overlap in roles between Social Worker, Health Visitor and Community Psychiatric Nurse. However, by 1972 70 per cent of Health Visitors and 68 per cent of District Nurses were working in association with general practitioners. At the same time, the pattern of Midwifery has become less rigid, 11 per cent of deliveries taking place at home whilst most

ante and post natal care took place in the community.[7] Thus, the
pattern of the Primary Health Care Team began to emerge, even though
in some rural areas some nurses are still functioning as Health Visitors,
School Nurses and District Nurses.

The number of Health Centres is growing, and the trend is for the
building of centres in large conurbations which are designed to promote
the integration of the team. Similarly the Consultative Document on
Priorities for Health and Social Services in England states that emphasis
should be given to encourage the development of Primary Health Care
Teams. As Health Centres emerge and Primary Health Care Teams
consolidate, occupational health nurses should find it easier to integrate
the care they give with the care given by these teams. Each Health
Centre should be made aware of the nature of the organisations for
which its clients/patients work and occupational health nurses should
take their place in the Primary Health Care team when this would
further the full recovery of the client/patient. This co-operation on the
part of the occupational health nurse might be especially useful where
the planning of care for the whole family is concerned and the Primary
Health Care Team is less able to assess the wage earner because that
person is at work and not easily available to the team.

The word team suggests harmony; each member of the Primary
Health Care Team brings a different training, experience and expertise.
The team normally consists of Health Visitors, District Nurses,
District Midwives, Social Workers, Community Psychiatric Nurses and
a General Practitioner. The team itself will need to liaise with other
health specialists when necessary. Occupational health nurses need to
recognise when they have a contribution to make to this team and in
order to do this they must be familiar with the changing roles of the
team members and the development of the teams within the Health
Centres with which they liaise. There will be times when they need an
involvement with a team member and times when they need to attend
case study conferences that involve a number of the team.

In a book of this nature, it is only possible to give a brief description
of the individual role of the nurses in the Primary Health Care Team.

The Health Visitor is a family visitor with expertise in child health
care and has a mandatory training. This training helps her to understand
relationships and the normal processes of growth and ageing. Like the
occupational health nurse, she too is concerned with the promotion of
health and the prevention of ill health through giving education, advice
and support and through the use of co-operation of outside agencies.
She visits families who may have no other regular contact with

health services and is leader of a team which can include SRNs, SENs and nursing auxiliaries who work in schools or clinics.

The school nurse is involved in the health supervision of school children and in the health education of children attending school. There is, at present, no mandatory training for school nurses. The trend in school health today is towards a system directed at the individual needs of each child which relies on school nurses, teachers and parents bringing the needs of the child to the attention of school doctors. Sometimes school nurses are closely associated with Health Visitors in the course of their routine work.

The District or Home Nurse is employed to give skilled nursing care to all persons living in the community. She may be leader of a team of SRNs or SENs and nursing auxiliaries. In the course of her work she too needs to constantly assess and reassess the needs of the patient and the family and liaise with members of the Primary Health Care Team and outside agencies as necessary. There is no mandatory training as yet for the District Nurse, although this may soon occur. Occupational health nurses may need to co-operate with District Nurses when treatment that has been available at work for patients needs to be continued at weekends or during holidays. Occupational health nurses may also have clients/patients with members of the family who need the attention of a District Nurse or Health Visitor.

Treatment room nurses can be employed by AHA, although this work can be undertaken by District Nurses (over and above their usual work). In either case these nurses undertake a wide variety of treatment in health centres or general practice premises.

Midwives have undergone statutory training and usually work in Midwifery Divisions. However, they can be involved in one or several Primary Health Care Teams for the provision of ante and post natal treatment and health education. They also attend at home confinements and may deliver mothers in hospital. Midwives are now becoming more involved in genetic counselling and family planning.

Practice nurses are employed by some general practitioners for nursing and/or reception duties. Sometimes they work alongside nurses employed by the NHS but they seldom give a treatment service outside the general practitioners' premises. This is the nurse that may well be involved with patients referred to the General Practitioner Service by occupational health nurses. It will be the practitioner who decides whether or not the OHN or the practice nurse continues the treatment. This is why it is so essential that the practitioner understands the qualifications and appreciates the level of competence of the occupational health nurse.

The Community Psychiatric Nurse is a Registered Mental Nurse who may be attached to a group practice, or a hospital service. Training for this fast growing nursing speciality is not mandatory but is becoming more easily obtainable through Joint Board of Clinical Nursing Studies (JBCNS) courses throughout the country. Community Psychiatric Nurses are mostly involved in the continuation of established care to patients who have been discharged from hospital. They have an advisory and supportive role to the family and are involved in socio-therapeutic techniques, such as behaviour therapy, psychotherapy and behaviour modification. It is hoped that the preventive aspects of the work will be developed when they all become community based.

The Nursing Officer is responsible for Health Visitors, midwives or District Nurses of her own discipline. This management structure was well described in *The Implementation of Mayston DHSS* (1973).[8] It is the responsibility of the Nursing Officer to be aware of the effectiveness of the team she leads.

A function of the Primary Health Care Team and its members is to liaise with the social work teams of the Local Authorities which will be described under LA services. Sometimes social workers are actually attached to a Primary Health Care Team and this in itself should improve communication.

Local Authority Services (LA)

Central government monitoring of this service is the responsibility of the Secretary of State for Health and Social Security. LA services are administered over most of the country by County Councils, in London by Borough Councils and in the greater provincial conurbations by Metropolitan District Councils. It is the responsibility of the LA to interpret current government policy and provide services locally. As in the NHS the delivery of services at local level will be affected by local motivation so that there is some variation in the distribution of quality and quantity of service throughout the country. Only those LA services that are co-ordinated with the NHS services and/or should be used by Occupational Health Services will be described here.

1. Environmental Health Services. Each LA provides an Environmental Health Service adminsitered by a Chief Officer who usually has the background of Senior Health Inspector. The Chief Officer has the benefit of advice and guidance from a Community Physician for those functions that relate to notifiable infectious diseases (e.g. food poisoning) and for this purpose, the Community Physician becomes a designated 'Proper Officer'. Whilst the Community Physician works for the Area Health Authority and often takes the title of Specialist in Community Health (Environmental Health, MOEH) he liaises between both authorities for the purpose of preventing and controlling outbreaks of notifiable infectious diseases. The occupational health nurse needs to understand the function of the MOEH, as she may be required to take part in any epidemiological investigation or programme for control of infection and work alongside the Environmental Health Inspectors (EHI) and Health Visitors when, for example, there is an outbreak of food poisoning which is traced to the food factory or works canteen for which the occupational health nurse has a responsibility. This apart, a thorough understanding of the Food and Hygiene (General) Regulations 1970 helps occupational health nurses co-operate with the EHI to ensure the regulations are implemented. EHI's have duties of inspection of some premises which are similar to those of the Health and Safety Inspectorate. Occupational health nurses may also meet the EHI when he visits the work place in connection with his duties under the Clean Air Act 1968.

2. Local Authority Social Service Department. Since the Secretary of State for Social Services is also responsible for the NHS he should be in a position to co-ordinate these services nationally and ensure that they develop in a balanced manner. However, when the Health and Social Service Departments amalgamated, the result was a huge unwieldy government department. Everyday practice is affected by the fact that the Social Service Departments are within the LA and not the NHS, and at district level, the LA Boundaries are not always coterminous with the NHS boundaries. This makes day-to-day communication and successful co-operation more difficult to achieve.

All major Local Authorities are required to provide comprehensive social services under the Local Authority Social Services Act 1970. This legislation followed the Seebohm Report of 1968.[9] Each authority has a Social Service Committee which controls the services and a Director of Social Services who administers the service.

The services provided by each Local Authority's Social Service Committee are listed to enable occupational health nurses to know to whom they can refer clients/patients who may require advice and care:

(a) care of the elderly;
(b) care of the physically handicapped including partially sighted,

deaf, spastics, epileptics and paraplegics;
(c)   care of the homeless;
(d)   child care protection;
(e)   social work and family casework;
(f)   care of children under five years;
(g)   the provision of home helps;
(h)   the care of unsupported mothers.

To effect integration between this department and the NHS there is a specialist in Community Medicine (Social Services) who like the MOEH is on the staff of the Area Medical Officer (NHS), but has the responsibility of giving medical advice as necessary to the social services.

Department of Education and Science

The Secretary of State for Education and Science is responsible to the government to see that the Education Acts and national policy are implemented. The three main stages of education for which the Local Authorities have responsibility are primary, secondary and tertiary education. Universities are within the realm of private education but receive finance from the government.

Occupational health nurses should be familiar with the provision of educational services generally and in particular with those which affect people at work. Parents may need to be advised about the Educational Welfare Service which deals with problems of absence from school, educational benefits, transport for those attending special schools and associated welfare benefits.

Whilst the overall responsibility for the Careers Service is vested in the Department of Employment, the services are directly provided by the Local Education Authority (LEA). These services are primarily for young people in education up to their point of entry to a first job. However, clients may return for advice at a later stage, and occupational health nurses may wish to make this known when counselling young people who have not made successful transitions from school to work. It is the Careers Office that employers have a duty to inform when they employ a young person.

Young people may also benefit from the Youth Service, the policy for which is laid down by the DES and provided by the LEA by the provision of informal educational and social activities for young people. Most LAs have Youth Committees advised by full time paid officers and attended by representatives of voluntary organisations.

Adult Education is based on local educational establishments, and catered for by the Workers' Educational Association, the extramural departments of universities and the Open University. Day and evening courses are offered. Many of these courses develop existing interests in hobbies etc., others prepare or offer training for redundant people or those wishing to return to work after a long absence (e.g. mothers) and there are useful courses which prepare people for retirement. Many people are still unaware of these courses which are attended predominantly by the middle classes and occupational health nurses could co-operate by reminding the people at work who show an interest in continuing education.

Voluntary Services

It is impossible and inappropriate to describe the many and varied voluntary services with which occupational health nurses should co-operate. It is better then, to assess the health and social problems that exist today and are predicted for the future and show how occupational health nurses may use voluntary services to complement statutory services. There are several up-to-date, inexpensive paperback books that outline voluntary services and should form part of the reference library of every occupational health department.

The HMSO publication *Prevention and Health: Everybody's Business*[10] reassesses public and personal health and in Chapter 3 current and future problems are identified as falling into three broad categories of disease: those associated with old age, those associated with man's behaviour and those relating to our changing environment.

Ischaemic heart disease, cancer and stroke constitute 66 per cent of all mortality in England and Wales. Ischaemic heart disease in men accounts for more years of productive life lost in those aged 15-64 years than any other single disease. The most important disease of women in this age group is cancer, with the emphasis on breast cancer. Strokes afflict both sexes in this age group whilst accidents and bronchitis are a problem in men. All these diseases can result in long term sickness absence and mortaility and, during this time, there may be a need to use several voluntary agencies to support either the sick person and/or his/her family. Industrial accidents and prescribed industrial diseases accounted for over 10 per cent of days lost by sickness in 1974. Those suffering serious accidents together with those suffering from prescribed industrial diseases may also need long-term support from voluntary as well as statutory services.

In 1971, 16 per cent of the population were of retirement age, and at present there are about 5 million people in the United Kingdom who are aged 65-74 years and a further 2.7 million of 75 years and over and 90 per cent of these live in their own home. It is predicted that in 25 years' time, the number over 75 years of age will increase by another .7 million in England and Wales. Since it is current NHS policy to keep (with the support of the Primary Health Care Team) these people at home rather than in institutions, it becomes apparent that the middle-aged children of these elderly people may be of working age and it may be that the problems that they experience are identified by occupational health nurses. Therefore, it is necessary to have a knowledge of those voluntary services that support the aged, services such as Age Concern, Women's Royal Voluntary Service, British Red Cross, Marie Curie Foundation and a knowledge of voluntary organisations which help people make a happy transition from work to retirement. It is difficult to assess the amount of disability that exists in the aged population, certainly defects affecting sight, hearing and mobility become increasingly common (e.g. 14,000 new cases of blindness are registered in Great Britain each year and 25 per cent of all people over 65 years suffer a significant degree of deafness and many need chiropody treatment to keep them mobile). The 1971 census showed that of the 8 million elderly people living in private households, about 2 million lived alone and, therefore, there must be problems of isolation and loneliness. Amelia Harris showed in 1971 that about ½ million women over 65 were handicapped and that of these, one-third lived alone. Other problems of old age are financial hardships and nutritional deficiencies. From these facts and figures it is easy to estimate that these problems will increase and that it is the voluntary services that help support the aged that may help occupational health nurses maintain the health and care of people who remain at work whilst caring for elderly relatives.

As yet, those diseases that result from the behaviour of individuals have been difficult to prevent, i.e. diseases related to smoking, alcoholism and drug dependence, obesity and the sexually transmitted diseases. Some employees will either be affected by these diseases themselves or have members of the family suffering from them. In both cases the employee concerned will suffer and may need support from the Occupational Health Department who, in turn, will advise the employee of the role and function of voluntary services that will co-operate to support both the individual and the family. Whilst smoking has tended to decline in men recently, smoking among wives of unskilled men is increasing and, as the number of smokers has decreased, those that continue to smoke are smoking more. The prevalence and the incidence of alcoholism continues to rise especially amongst women [11] and young people.[12] There are several agencies that will co-operate to overcome this problem, such agencies as Alcoholics Anonymous and Al Anon which supports the family too. The misuse of drugs can result in addiction and self-poisoning. The Samaritans are one of the agencies that may prove invaluable to the client/patient with suicidal tendencies.

As women have changed their smoking and drinking habits, so they have changed their attitudes to sex: advances in contraception and abortion services have largely safe-guarded against unwanted pregnancy. However, with the trend towards early marriage and the high divorse rate, it may be that more young people need the help of the National Marriage Guidance Council, who are willing to counsel couples before marriage as well as to help resolve marital problems.

The Finer Report 1974,[13] drew attention to the needs of single-parent families; many of these parents are at work and may welcome an introduction to 'Gingerbread' which is an association of one-parent families, in other words, a self-help group whose members consist of divorced, separated, widowed, unmarried, prison spouses and parents who have severely disabled partners.

Children of working parents can experience problems and the problems are often discussed with the occupational health nurse. There are many voluntary services for children of all ages, ranging from those who take children into care, like those who have residential schools for physically handicapped, emotionally subnormal children, as well as play schemes, baby sitters, day centres and holiday schemes, to those who organise social activities like the Scouts and Guide movement and the youth groups attached to many churches.

About ½ million immigrants from the New Commonwealth have entered the United Kingdom in the past ten years. The 1971 census revealed 46,000 immigrants born on the Indian sub-continent, 300,000 born in the West Indies, 7 million immigrants of Irish origin and another 1 million from other countries. Occupational health nurses having immigrant groups in the working population need to co-operate with the NHS in health supervision for these groups who present with specific problems and also ensure that the psycho-social strain on immigrants is reduced by making them aware of organisations that specialise in their problems.

A national policy that aims at the early resettlement of the mentally ill and mentally handicapped in the community means that there is an increasing need to be aware of voluntary services that offer care and support to individuals and to families.

There are many more health and social problems, that have not been mentioned here since individually these problems have not, in themselves, reached national proportions. Examples of these are chronic diseases like epilepsy and multiple sclerosis; there are a variety of voluntary services directed at relieving the suffering of individuals and families who need help.

The third category of problems, those that relate to the physical environment and disease, draws attention to the effect of the environment in which we live and the environment in which we work. It has been said that industry is a provider of Social Services,[14] private Occupational Health Services are voluntary services and benefit is obtained if Occupational Health Services co-operate with each other.

In conclusion, co-operation will be achieved when each person that is involved in a 'caring system' is trained in his or her speciality, understands his or her individual role, appreciates his or her strengths and weaknesses, receives continuous education and is prepared to accept that there will be times when roles overlap and that there is a continuous need to understand how colleagues complement and supplement teamwork, especially when there is no manager directly responsible for the team's performance.

Notes

1. P. Friend, 'Nursing in Primary Care', *Nursing Mirror* (14 July 1977), p.41.

2. The Future of Voluntary Organisations: Report of the Wolfenden Committee (Croom Helm, London, 1978).

3. M. Young and P. Willmott, *The Symmetrical Family* (Routledge and Kegan Paul, London, 1973), p.65.

4. S. Gauvain, *Occupational Health: a Guide to Sources of Information* (Heinemann, London, 1974).

5. Safety Representatives and Safety Committee Regulations. Statutory Instrument, no. 500 (HMSO, London, 1977).

6. Occupations and Conditions of Work (HMSO, London, 1976), p.4.

7. For further details see R. Levitt, *The Reorganised National Health Service*, 2nd edn. (Croom Helm, London, 1977).

8. Department of Health and Social Security, *Management Structure in the Local Authority Nursing Services: the Implementation of Mayston* (HMSO, London, 1973).

9. F. Seebohm, Report of the Committee on Local Authority and Allied Social Services (HMSO, London, 1968).

10. Department of Health and Social Security, *Prevention and Health: Everybody's Business* (HMSO, London, 1976).

11. A Harris, *Social Welfare for the Elderly*, Government Social Survey (HMSO, London, 1971).